T0317379

Wild Medicine

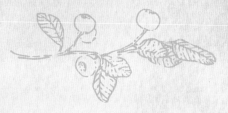

An Illustrated Guide to the Magick of Herbs

Shelby Bundy & Kate Belew

Paintings by Zarina Karapetyan

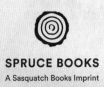

SPRUCE BOOKS

A Sasquatch Books Imprint

To Jason, Saylor, and Chase:
For always letting me grow wild. I love you.
—Shelby

To and for the plants.
With gratitude to my family, parents,
siblings, Cody and Banjo, and my teachers.
This is for (and because of) you.
xo, Kate

Printed in China

SPRUCE BOOKS with colophon is a registered trademark
of Penguin Random House LLC

28 27 26 25 24 23   9 8 7 6 5 4 3 2 1

Editor: Sharyn Rosart | Production editor: Peggy Gannon
Herb paintings: Zarina Karapetyan
Botanical spot art: © Ekaterina / Adobe Stock | Celestial spot art: © Venimo / Adobe Stock
Moon phase spot art: © Handdraw / Adobe Stock

ISBN: 978-1-63217-497-0

Spruce Books, a Sasquatch Books Imprint
1325 Fourth Avenue, Suite 1025, Seattle, WA 98101

SasquatchBooks.com

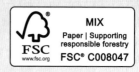

MIX
Paper | Supporting
responsible forestry
FSC® C008047
FSC
www.fsc.org

Contents

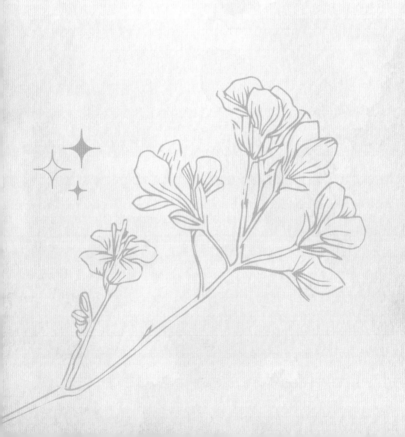

List of Herbs

Bay
Blackberry
Black Cohosh
Boneset
Burdock
Calendula
Cayenne
Chamomile, German
Chickweed
Chrysanthemum
Clary Sage
Cleavers
Comfrey
Crampbark
Damiana
Dandelion
Echinacea
Elder
Elecampane
Eucalyptus
Fennel
Feverfew
Ginger
Goldenrod
Goldenseal
Gotu Kola
Gumweed
Hawthorn
Hibiscus
Holy Basil
Hyssop

Jasmine
Juniper Berry
Lady's Mantle
Lavender
Lemon Balm
Lemongrass
Linden
Marshmallow
Meadowsweet
Motherwort
Mugwort
Mullein
Nettle
Oatstraw
Oregano
Passionflower
Peppermint
Pipsissewa
Plantain
Red Clover
Rose
Rosemary
Slippery Elm
Skullcap
St. John's Wort
Turmeric
Valerian
Vitex
White Willow
Witch Hazel
Yarrow
Yellow Dock

Preface

Both of us found green magick out of necessity.

In a world that so frequently tries to separate us from our essential connection to the land and all the life it nourishes, it can be a challenge to stay connected. There are so many obstacles—the constant sense of urgency and innumerable deadlines that add up to the hectic demands of so-called modern life—not to mention the physical distance that often separates us from the natural world, which may be due to our living situations being disconnected from nature, a scarcity of green spaces, especially in urban areas, or just the daily busyness that prevents us from even seeing the life around us. Despite all of it, the plants are still there, waiting for each of us to make our way back to them.

Through daily ritual, gardening, getting dirt under our fingernails, apprenticeships, reading books, studying with experts, and learning by doing, eventually we both answered the call—and continue to answer it, again and again. The plants want us to succeed, and we owe it to them to do so.

This book is a collaboration between two writers, witches, and friends. Back in 2016, Shelby Bundy started building an apothecary, and began guiding her friends and family through working with wild medicine; the Tamed Wild community you see today grew from her efforts. More recently, Kate Belew joined Shelby on this journey, bringing her skills as a storyteller, herbalist, and writer to Tamed Wild.

This book began as two unique and beautifully illustrated card decks created to support the study of wild medicine by providing an easy-to-use reference guide to the major healing herbs (dreamed up by Shelby after finding nothing like it on the market years ago!). Over time we added layers of lore and wisdom, along with full-blown spells, rituals, and stories—and created this very book you now hold in your hands.

These pages are full of learnings from our own herbal journeys, and we hope they will support you on yours. For as many herbalists as you can gather in a room, there will always be as many opinions, stories, and

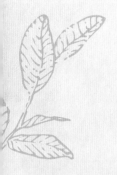

experiences to share about each of these plants. And that's one of the great gifts of green medicine—the honoring of individual experience.

We hope you will get to know these plants as we have, and continue to gain knowledge as you go. The journey is rewarding—and accompanied by many plant friends. We'll see you out there.

Magickally,
Shelby Bundy and Kate Belew

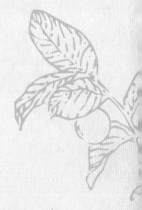

Shelby's Plant Story

How does anyone find their way back to nature? For me, it was necessity.

My path to green witchery began in 2016 when I was told that my then-eight-year-old daughter was struggling in school and showing symptoms of ADD. While I believed her teachers were having this experience with her, her dad and I saw no signs of it at home. We were put off by how quickly we were told to take her to the doctor and put her on medication. When asked what her problematic behaviors looked like, they told us, "she looks out the window a lot," "can't stay focused," and "daydreams." While not paying attention in a school environment is not ideal, did looking out the window really require a doctor's intervention? We were hesitant to medicate the dreamer out of her. Surely there was another way? Thus began my journey into Wild Medicine.

I enrolled in an herbalism course and turned the old carriage house of my one-hundred-year-old home into an apothecary. I spent my evenings learning all I could about the traditional healing properties of herbs, while brewing and blending by hand all the while. When my daughter came home from school, we would test out the new blends to find the perfect "homework tea" that would help her focus and stay on task. In the mornings before school, we would try another blend with breakfast, and I would send her off with a rollerball full of essential oils for a midday pick-me-up.

I became obsessed and began crafting "replacements" for commonly used items in our medicine cabinet—salves for scrapes, cough syrups and drops, herbal steams for cold and allergy season. We found that not only did they work as well as or better than their commercial pharmaceutical counterparts, but in making and using these remedies, we were forming a deep connection with the plants in the process.

We kept investigating, and later that year we learned our daughter's symptoms were not in fact from ADD, but a result of her having been born completely deaf in her left ear! It was a surprise, as she had passed her hearing tests up to that point. Moreover, her "daydreamer" personality was among the things we loved most about her. Classrooms were difficult environments for her because she couldn't always hear the teacher, and the noise of multiple children talking would make it difficult for her decipher what was being said. Therefore, she looked out the window and doodled on her papers, much like children with ADD may do. In her case, the medication would never have been an effective treatment.

By that time, however, the teas we created together had become an important little ritual for us and an essential and fun part of our day. We had a renewed connection to each other and to nature. The path toward healing her ended up healing all of us in ways I cannot fully articulate. It changed my family, and it changed me—not only in the way I look at plants and the living world, but by making me realize there was a way to live differently. It paved the way for me to create Tamed Wild, and to meet Kate Belew, who became a cherished friend and cowriter, and it eventually led me to write this book. It came back to the plants, which provided me with an awakening and an opportunity I didn't even know I needed.

Necessity. What do you need?

Maybe you live in a city where the unending bustle of busy streets has you yearning for open fields and leafy paths. Perhaps you've wondered whether you should pack up and move to the countryside—or maybe just plant yourself a balcony garden. Possibly you live near nature but your job requires hours upon hours of sitting in front of a computer and you realize you are out of balance with what lives outside your office window. Or perhaps, for the sake of your mental health, your doctor is telling you to "get outside for a walk" or "spend some time in nature."

Whatever necessity brought you here, welcome to this path. Know that it will be full of brambles and thorns, flowers and roots, lush springs and barren winters. That is the way of Wild Medicine, and that is the beauty of this journey.

I am honored to be on it with you, magickal one.
—Shelby Bundy

Kate's Plant Story

Hello Wild One,

Plant medicine and magick are potent portals.

My journey with plants has been meandering and vine-like. I grew up in a small town in southwest Michigan, a block from my grandparents' house. Both my mom and grandma kept gardens, and I remember spending time there and learning from my family members about the plants they grew in these green spaces.

There was also wild space—the forest behind the house that was my playground, the beginning of my imagination, and the place I found solace in the world.

Queen Anne's lace, oak, birch, and cedar were some of my first friends.

As I grew up, I continued my relationship with plants through the practice of writing. I have always been a writer, so it was natural for these worlds to wind, weave, and intersect.

Through those early years of studying after leaving my hometown, I read poems that gave voice to nature and allowed me, through story, to return to that creative source, the fecundity, the fertile earth.

Inspired by Federico Garcia Lorca's concept of *duende*, a concept taken from folklore and developed into a theory of creative works, and with the guidance of my mentor, poet Diane Seuss, my relationship with the natural world flourished. I deepened my experience, knowing that plants are poetry, living in this world. "All that has dark sounds has duende."

Plants and perhaps duende brought me to New York City, and in the aisles of apothecaries, in the digital realm, inside the secrets of the sacred written word, and in the classroom, I learned—and I became more and more myself with each adventure and each new lesson.

The plants led me to my herbal apprenticeship with wise woman and Green Witch Robin Rose Bennett. Plants crafted a wild world for me. And with their guidance, I return to the mountains of the East Coast, the rural-ness and the memories of where I grew up, and listen to the messages of the old hills, fields, roots, weeds, and all that resists and is untamed.

I met Shelby Bundy through our mutual love of plants. Since 2020, I have worked with her at Tamed Wild, telling stories, weaving worlds, and shar-ing messages from plants as a cohost on the podcast *Magick & Alchemy* and as a writer for the blog, social media, herbal publications, rituals, gri-moire pages, and decks that Shelby has dreamed up. This book that you're holding in your hands is one of the projects she invited me to support her on, so I brought all my love of plants to these pages with that intention.

Plants remind me that we are not separate from nature; we are nature ourselves. Plants have been my lifelong companions, and I will be a stu-dent of their lessons and messages forever. Maybe you're new on this path of the Green Witch, or maybe it's one you've been walking for a while. These journeys are sometimes complicated, with surprising rocks or turns, but also with that beautiful, dappled light shining through the trees. No matter where you are on your journey, I'm so glad we're crossing paths here, sharing our love of herbs and wild medicine.

I hope these musings and pieces of inspiration I've gathered along the way serve you as they have served me.

To the plants and to your beautiful, wild wholeness.

xo,
Kate

How to Work with Plants

Tea

A beautiful and easy way to work with herbs is to brew them into a cup of tea. This can be done with a strainer, reusable tea bags, or disposable tea bags. You can blend mixtures of herbs, add boiling water, allow the mixture to steep, and then sip away! Different herbs have different steeping times, so as you get to know the plants, you'll get to know the ideal amount of time to brew your favorite cup. Teas are a marvelous way to bring herbs into your daily rituals. They are delicious, affordable, and supportive, providing a pause for quiet contemplation or shared enjoyment.

Infusion

An infusion is a wonderful way to receive the nutrients of the plants and herbs you're working with. The first step is deciding whether it will be hot or cold. Some herbs respond better to cold infusions, others to hot infusions, so you'll want to assess your herbs and your intention before deciding (for example, mucilaginous herbs respond better to cold water!). For a hot infusion, add herbs to a boil-safe container such as a mason jar (be careful that the jar isn't cold, because adding hot liquid can cause it to crack!). Then, boil your water and pour it over the herbs in the jar. Cover the mixture with a lid to keep volatile oils in, but don't overtighten—it's better to keep a little bit of give. Allow the jar to sit in the refrigerator for a period of time. Some herbs are best left overnight, while others need only a few hours. With time and experimentation, you'll discover what works best. When the infusion is ready, strain the mixture, pressing out the plant material to release the fullest amount of nutrients. Don't throw away the spent herbs—compost the plant matter to return it to the earth. (Note that some plants can be used in a second infusion.) Get to know your plants and try an infusion—they're delicious. Drink them much like a tea! (That is, a tea with more nutrients packed in.)

Tincture or Glycerite

A tincture or glycerite is a method of preparing plant-based medicine that uses a solvent like vodka, brandy, vinegar, or glycerin to extract nutrients from the plant. There are a few different methods of tincture making, but the kind that I'm most familiar with is the folk method. First, depending on what you have on hand, decide whether you will be using fresh or dried herbs. Next, macerate the herbs, which entails chopping them up to help the tincturing process along. Take your fresh or dried herbs and fill a mason-type jar ½ to ⅔ full of the plant material. Then, pour your solvent over the plants, filling the jar to the top. Store the jar in a dark and dry place for six weeks, shaking it every couple of days. The final step is to decant the tincture: strain the mixture through clean cheesecloth, squeezing out the plant material before pouring the mixture into dropper bottles. If your process calls for a more exact method, you may want to learn the weight method of making a tincture. We don't cover that here, but you can find explanations online or in study with a more experienced herbalist.

Elixir

An elixir is created the same way as a tincture, but with a touch of added sweetness, ideally from honey! This is delicious and works especially well with plants like elderberry.

Infused Oil

To make a plant-infused oil, first select your herb(s) and an oil—olive, sunflower, and jojoba are a few favorites. If the herbs are fresh, allow them to dry for one or two days, because water in the oil will cause mold to grow. Fill the jar with plant material, and then cover it with oil. Before sealing the jar, poke out any air bubbles. Check it regularly, and as it settles, you may want to top off the jar with more oil. Leave it in a cool, dark place for four to six weeks, then strain into jars. Squeeze the plant material to get out all the nutrients, then return it to the earth.

Salve

For a salve, you will first make an herb-infused oil, as described on the previous page. You'll need a glass jar, and either beeswax or shea butter. You will also need a double boiler for this preparation method. (If you don't have one on hand, the internet has loads of creative ideas for rigging one up yourself.) When the oil is ready to decant, boil down the beeswax or shea, then stir in the oil. You'll want to make a tester first to make sure the ratios are correct—do this by filling one of your jars and putting it in the freezer for a few minutes, then see if the texture is what you want.

Decoction

A decoction is simply a tea that is simmered. This process is frequently called upon when using bark and roots. Using a stovetop-safe pot (made of glass or stainless steel), place the herbs in the water, bring it to a boil, then simmer the mixture for twenty minutes. When the preparation is ready, strain, squeeze the materials, and then sip!

Syrup

When they said that "a spoonful of sugar helps the medicine go down," they were talking about herbal syrups. To make one, prepare a strong decoction and simmer it down to half of its volume, then add honey to taste. Allow the syrup to cool, then store it in a dark bottle. These can be kept for six months (the perfect amount of time to last through winter).

Honey

You can infuse herbs into honey to make a tasty delivery system for herbal medicine. A favorite infusion of ours is garlic in honey, which is perfect for the winter months. Add your plant material to a jar, and cover with honey. Allow it to steep for four to six weeks, and then enjoy. Reminder: young children (less than twelve months old) shouldn't have honey, as they are at risk from bacteria that can cause a very serious condition called infant botulism.

And More!

There are many other wonderful ways to work with herbs. Some herbalists feel called by flower essences, some by medicinal and ritual baths. There are fire ciders, which come in many varieties and can be a great way to work with culinary herbs in medicine. Vinegars are a delicious way to infuse medicine. Some herbalists craft scrubs, plant-based makeup, and more. Experiment with the plants you feel most called to and then see what they teach you. Listening to plants is step number one for making plant magick! To help you get started, we have included suggestions for each of the herbs in this book, including small ritual ideas and recipes. While reading about herbs and plant magick is fun and potent, actually getting dirt under your fingernails and working with the plants is the best way to learn.

Gathering Plants

When gathering plants, it's important to do it mindfully, paying attention to your actions, choices, and impact on the environment. Research to learn which plants in your area are at risk or endangered; there are websites like United Plant Savers that provide up-to-date information. You'll want to gather in a place that hasn't been sprayed for pesticides, on land that you're familiar with. There are many look-alike plants, with some of the look-alikes being toxic. Before gathering plants, gain as much knowledge as you can. Find an expert local plant identifier, or go for a weed walk with a knowledgeable herbalist or gardener. It's best to get to know the plants intimately before gathering them for yourself.

Another way to learn about plants is to grow and cultivate them yourself. Keeping a garden is a special way to tend to your relationship with the natural world. I was taught to do the best you can with what you've got, so when purchasing herbs, buy the best that you can afford (organic, etc.) and support trusted, small, local shops whenever you can. The happier and better tended the herbs, the better the medicine.

Asking Permission

Before gathering from a plant, it's important to ask the plant permission. Approach respectfully and quietly. Notice in your body what a "yes" and a "no" sound like. And even if you don't understand at first why you've heard a "no" from a specific plant or herb, trust that nature has reasons.

The Importance of Reciprocity

I was taught to be in reciprocal relationship with the herbs that I gather from, trying to give back and not just take. This might mean leaving a bit of dried herbs as an offering to the plant; offering something of yourself, such as a tear or a hair; or even reading a poem or a prayer—sharing whatever is sacred or meaningful to you. Know that the plants can feel your gratitude and sense your presence. Develop relationships of reciprocity with the plants and trees on your land and they'll be glad to see you each day—and, happily, this feeling is contagious.

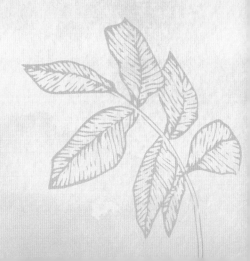

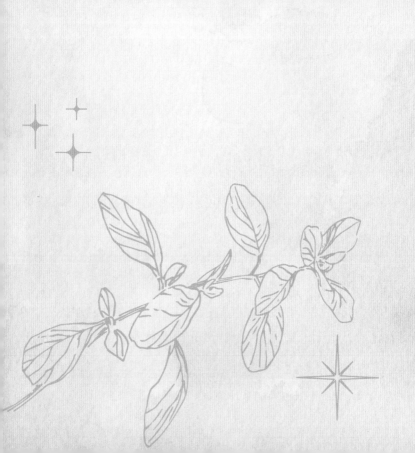

The
Herbs

Bay

Laurus nobilis

The Wishing Leaf

Bay leaf is an aromatic leaf that grows on several slow-growing species of trees known as bay laurel, California bay, sweet bay, or simply laurel. These trees are native to Asia and have been cultivated since ancient times throughout the Mediterranean.

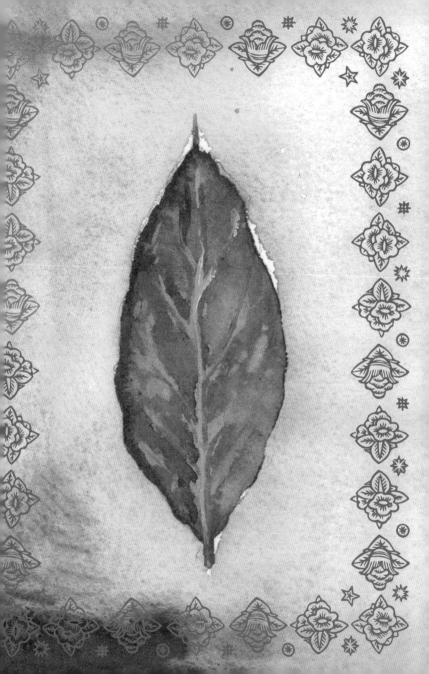

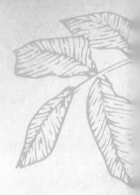

Parts Used: Leaves

Historical Medicinal Uses: Historically, in herbal medicine, bay leaf was used to treat wounds and as a soothing salve. Bay leaf is also a traditional culinary seasoning in many cultures, used to flavor soups, stews, and stocks.

How to Use: Leaf, oil, powder

Lore: In Greek mythology, the mountain nymph Daphne, fleeing from the advances of the god Apollo, changed into a laurel tree, which was forever after associated with Apollo. In ancient Rome, laurel wreaths were worn to symbolize power, victory, and prosperity.

Magickal Uses: In magick, work with bay leaves to craft spells for manifestation, prosperity, cleansing, and psychic development. It can also be helpful with wishes. It is said that in ancient Greece, the priestesses of Apollo would chew bay leaves or inhale the burning fumes of bay to induce prophetic visioning.

Easy Rituals, Potions, and Recipes: To manifest a wish with a bay leaf, purchase a dried leaf (you can find these in the spices section of the supermarket). Then, with a pen, write your wish, your intention, and what you're planning to manifest on the leaf itself (you'll have to keep it short to fit on the leaf). After you write your wish, hold the leaf in both of your hands, envisioning the intention as if it has already come to be. What does it feel like? Sound like? Taste like? Use all of your available senses. Then, once you feel ready, burn the bay leaf (safely) and watch the smoke carry your wish away. After burning, work together with the forces of the universe to live into this new reality.

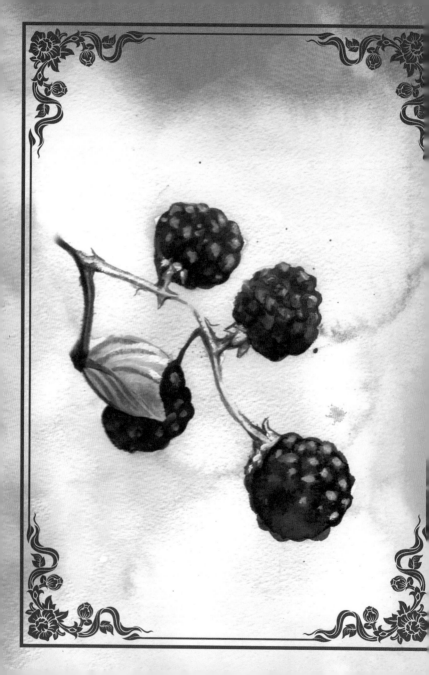

BLACKBERRY

Rubus villosus

The Protector

Blackberry is a bramble plant that grows 5–8 feet (1.5–2.4 m) tall. It contains single shrubs growing up to 8 feet (2.4 m) wide, and is often found in thickets, that is, growing through the middle of other plants. Thorny canes grow to produce a white flower with 3 to 5 petals and a berry that is deep-violet to black in color.

Parts Used: Leaves, root, bark, berries

Historical Medicinal Uses: Dating back over two thousand years, medicine made from the blackberry plant has been hailed as a cough suppressant and fever reducer, as well as a treatment for lung infections, bowel issues, bug bites, and boils. The berries are packed with vitamin C (a well-known antioxidant), and the leaves can be made into a tea that helps soothe a sore throat.

How to Use: Tea, tincture, poultice; culinary uses

Lore: When collected under certain phases of the moon, blackberries were believed to protect against spells, curses, and other spiritual attacks; they were used in this way in ritual. The thorny bushes were often planted around European villages and homes to protect against intruders and enemies. Some believe that the biblical burning bush shown to Moses was a blackberry bush.

Magickal Uses: Use blackberry on your altar—clip a piece of branch or pick some berries to put in a bowl as an offering to Brighid, the Celtic triple goddess of springtime and fertility. Place clippings from the thorny brambles near thresholds to protect the premises from negative energies.

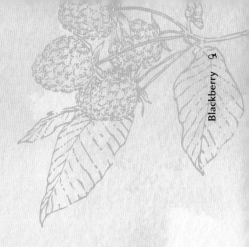

Easy Rituals, Potions, and Recipes: Create a magickal intention letter with the leaves and berries of the blackberry bush by pressing them onto paper and writing with the berry ink. Simply pluck the berries and leaves from their stems, thanking them for their offering in your magickal workings. Crush the berries in a mortar and pestle until you have a liquid or juice-like consistency. Using a quill pen or stick from the bramble, write your intentions on a piece of paper. Do not worry about the neatness or clarity, you are simply infusing your intentions through the berry ink. You can draw lines, symbols, or string together words—it does not matter. When you are finished, take the leaves and press them onto the berry-stained paper. Fold the paper three times, with the leaves inside. Depending on your intentions, you can burn the letter in a candle while "letting go" of that which is written, or bury it beneath a blackberry bramble to plant your intentions for future growth.

BLACK COHOSH

Cimicifuga racemosa

The Midwives' Herb

Black cohosh has deep-green, fernlike leaves that are tri-divided, complete with three-lobed terminal leaflets. Of the sharply toothed leaflets, look for the middle leaf to present itself as the largest. It can grow 3–8 feet (1–2.4 m) in height, sending up tall shoots of white flowers. It is also known as snakeroot, black bugbane, rattleweed, or rheumatism weed.

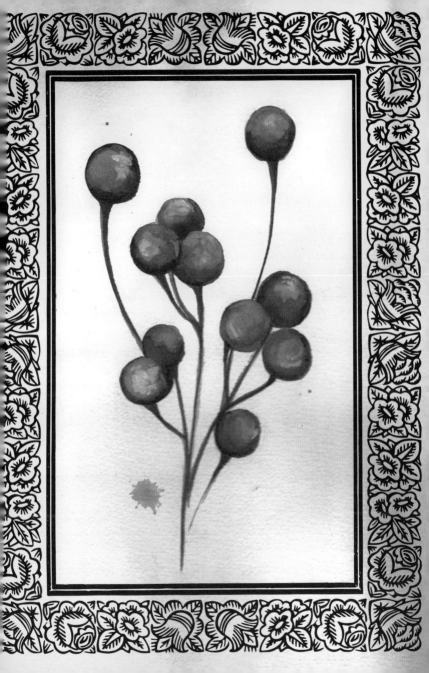

Parts Used: Root, rhizome

Historical Medicinal Uses: Black cohosh has a history of being an effective plant medicine for uterine support, and was often used to ease the pain of menstrual cramps and reduce hot flashes in menopause. To this day, black cohosh is used to treat menopausal symptoms (including hot flashes). It is also used to reduce inflammation in those who suffer from rheumatism and arthritis.

How to Use: Decoction, tincture, capsule

Lore: Black cohosh is also known as snakeroot for its ability to help heal snakebites. Indigenous peoples in North America also found great value in the use of black cohosh (alongside blue cohosh) in pregnancy and labor. Used early in pregnancy, it was known to be effective in terminating pregnancy or expelling tissue after a miscarriage. Taken during full-term labor, black cohosh was given to regulate contractions, restart stalled labor, and strengthen the uterus. Some midwives today continue to use the herb this way.

Magickal Uses: In magickal practice, black cohosh can be used to work with the archetypes of the goddess and the crone. Black cohosh has deep womb knowledge and can be helpful in rituals relating to fertility.

Easy Rituals, Potions, and Recipes: Sprinkle pieces of black cohosh into an offering bowl to the Crone Goddess before requesting her wisdom.

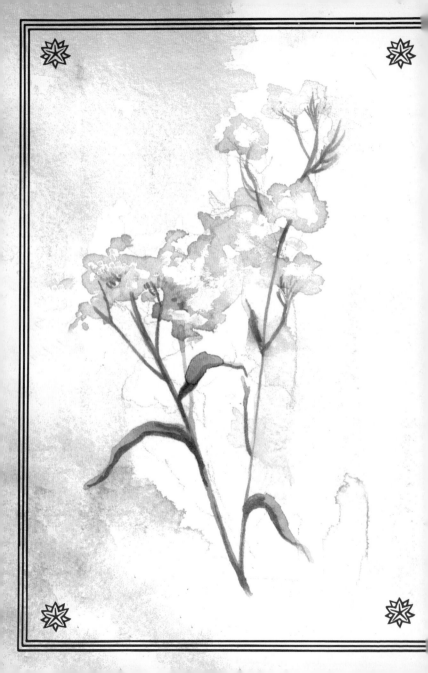

BONESET

Eupatorium perfoliatum

The Sweating Plant

Boneset is usually found growing in wetlands; its hairy, rough stems reach straight up to about 5 feet (1.5 m). Boneset plants are recognizable by their white clusters of flowers and leaves with long, pointed tips. Native to North America, boneset is a member of the aster family.

Parts Used: Leaves

Historical Medicinal Uses: Boneset has a long history of medicinal use by Indigenous peoples in North America. Those who ingested boneset reported the herb relieved pain in their bones that accompanied a flu-like illness they called "break-bone fever." In American folk medicine, this aromatic and bitter herb was traditionally simmered with honey and lemon to a make cough syrup that was used during the flu epidemic of 1918.

How to Use: Infusion, tincture, glycerite, wash

Lore: It is said that burning boneset in your home will drive away ghosts and unwanted spirits. The leaves are said to draw curses out of the body when they are rubbed on the skin, then burned in a fire.

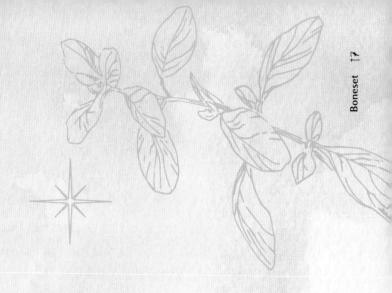

Magickal Uses: Boneset is known magickally for its protective prowess against unwanted spirits. Sprinkle a bit of dried boneset or boneset leaves on your windowsills or doorframes, or swirl it into a floor wash to banish negative presences and to help cleanse, clear, and break curses.

Easy Rituals, Potions, and Recipes: Harvest the leaves and flowers of a boneset plant, or purchase them from a trusted and local source. Using a mortar and pestle, crush up the leaves and flowers while imagining that any negative energy directed at you is being deflected away and returned to those who sent it. Mix crushed boneset with a bit of salt and keep it in a dish near your doors and windows to act as plant magick protection. After one moon cycle, return the salt and boneset to running water and imagine allowing yourself to return to a state of flow.

BURDOCK

Arctium lappa

Beggar's Buttons

Burdock is a tall plant that many call a weed. Reaching 9 feet (2.7 m) in height, the lower part of the burdock plant has large leaves with short gray hairs on their undersides. Smaller leaves adorn the upper part of the plant, along with clusters of purple flowers with hooked bracts. During the first year of growth, it displays only leaves; in the second, the tall stalks appear, topped with purple flowers and burrs.

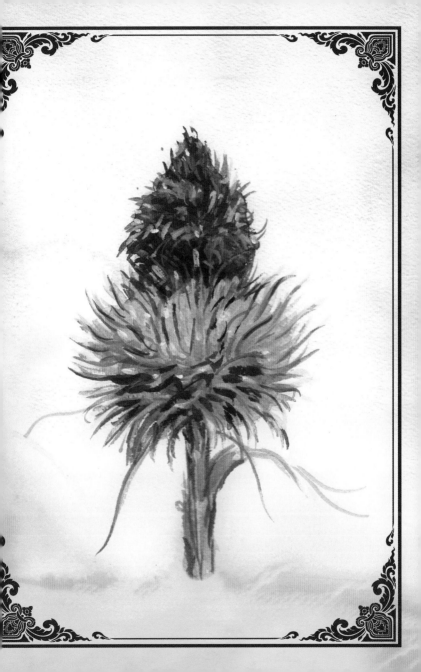

Parts Used: Leaves, root, seeds

Historical Medicinal Uses: Historically known as a blood purifier and digestive aid, burdock's bitter actions make it popular among herbalists for moving things along in the digestive tract. It has also been known as a topical skin treatment for acne, and a wrinkle reducer.

How to Use: Decoction, tincture, ingestion

Lore: Some believe that the Fae ride horses around under cover of the night and braid their hair, tangling the strands with burdock burrs. The Swiss engineer George de Mestral invented Velcro after examining the fruit of a burdock plant that had stuck to his dog's fur.

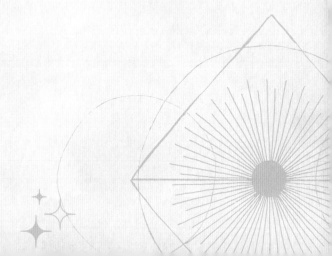

Magickal Uses: The burdock plant is used as a protective herb. In rituals, keep burdock root close to help dispel negative energy, and as a supportive plant. Sprinkle any part of the plant around your home and sacred spaces to create a protective border between your world and any harmful energies from the outside world.

Easy Rituals, Potions, and Recipes: Create a tincture of burdock root to drop into your tea as a digestive aid. Place the root in a jar, filling it ⅔ of the way. Cover with vodka and close the lid. Store in a dark cupboard for one moon cycle, or thirty days. Strain the liquid and thank the roots for their work as a plant ally. Return the spent roots to the earth and place the liquid into a dropper bottle. You can take it directly from the dropper or add a few drops to your evening tea.

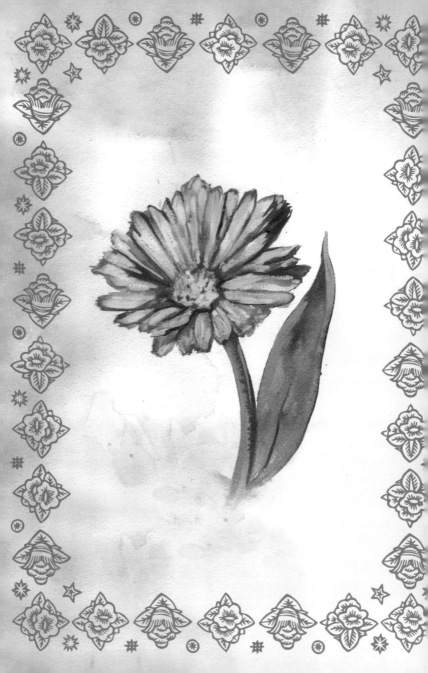

CALENDULA

Calendula officinalis

The Sunshine Herb

Calendula can be easily identified due to its bright-orange blossoms. A member of the daisy family, calendula is also known as pot marigold, common marigold, or Scotch marigold. Flower petals are orange to deep yellow with a 1–3 inch (2.5–7.6 cm) central cluster of tubular flowers, surrounded by several rows of ray florets. The stalk can grow up to 2 feet (61 cm) tall and produces stems with medium-green leaves covered in small hairlike strands.

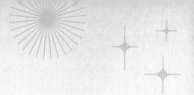

Parts Used: Flowers, florets

Historical Medicinal Uses: Known for its bright and sunny personality, calendula has long been hailed as potent plant medicine. Said to detoxify the liver and gallbladder, calendula petals have a historical reputation as an effective topical aid for cuts, scrapes, burns, and bites. The dried petals are also commonly used in tea blends as well as tinctures. Infused into a carrier oil, calendula can be added to butters and balms to create salves. It has also been used in soups and stews as an immune-boosting ingredient.

How to Use: Infusion, tea, tincture, salve, and balm

Lore: Calendula has been used in rituals for centuries. The ancient Greeks and Romans wore calendula crowns, and Hindu peoples used it to decorate statues of deities. Calendula is still found today adorning Day of the Dead altars in Mexico and Central America. Lore has it that if you cast a handful of calendula petals across your bed, you will be safe and protected. It was also said that calendula could offer prophetic dreams.

Magickal Uses: The whole blossoms of calendula, and even its petals, can offer us the generous brightness of blessed days. Keep calendula in your pocket when you're trying to stay on the sunny side of life, and allow its energy to move stagnated flow.

Easy Rituals, Potions, and Recipes: Soak in the energy of calendula by adding some of her bright petals to your bathwater. Simply add a scoop of petals to a mesh tea strainer or cheesecloth sachet and toss in the water. (This keeps your drain from becoming clogged!) Slip into the water and close your eyes. Take a few deep breaths and envision the positive energy of the calendula-infused water cleansing away any negativity you may be holding. Picture the orange and yellow colors of the petals reaching into all the darkness you may be carrying, illuminating those spaces with glowing light. When you have completed your bathing ritual, unplug the drain, allowing the negative energies to leave with the water. Take your used calendula petals to the garden or another patch of soil. Whisper gratitude for their assistance, and return them to the earth.

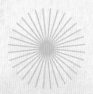

CAYENNE

Capsicum annuum

The Spicy Herb

Cayenne is a shrublike plant with small, off-white, sometimes purple-tinted flowers that typically grow in groups of five. It has elliptical-shaped leaves with smooth edges. The fruit produced (peppers) can be red, yellow, or green when ripe.

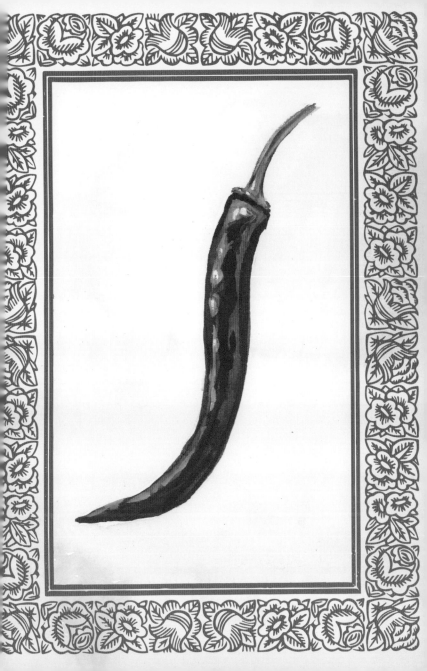

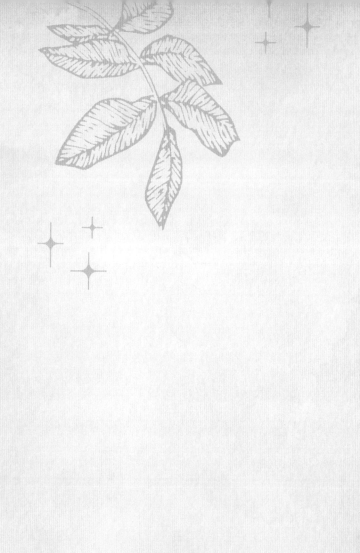

Parts Used: Fruit (pepper), leaves

Historical Medicinal Uses: Not only is it a wildly popular culinary plant renowned for its ability to spice up any dish, cayenne also has a reputation as a powerful aphrodisiac. Historically, it has been used most to relieve headache pain, reduce fever, and treat sinus issues.

How to Use: Ingestion

Lore: Cayenne peppers were used in Aztec rituals to ward off evil entities. Popular with folk healers throughout history as a protective herb, they were commonly worn as a necklace or, in powdered form, could be sprinkled around one's home.

Magickal Uses: Cayenne peppers can be ground into powder form to sprinkle on candles during love spells. Add cayenne to sex magick spells to increase the "fire" and passion.

Easy Rituals, Potions, and Recipes: For an easy passion spell, simply write your desires on a piece of paper and fold it three times. With a piece of ribbon or string, tie the paper to a cayenne pepper while whispering your intent. Bury it in your garden near a rose bush for a touch of love.

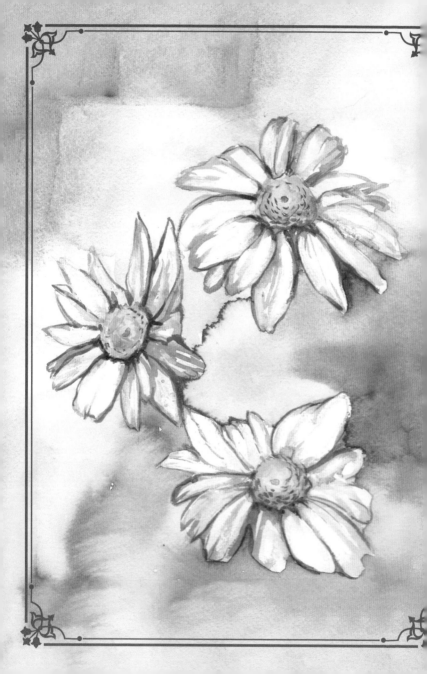

CHAMOMILE, GERMAN

Matricaria recutita

The Children's Herb

Chamomile got its name from the Greek words meaning "ground" and "apple" because the plant grows low to the ground and has a sweet smell. You can recognize chamomile by its delicate, small flowers with puffy yellow centers and small, elongated white petals that grow downward away from the center. Chamomile can grow 6-24 inches (15-61 cm) tall.

Parts Used: Flower head

Historical Medicinal Uses: Chamomile is a well-known and loved herb among healers, and its medicinal properties were documented by the ancient Greeks, Romans, and Egyptians. It has been used as a bitter to treat digestive and stomach issues, including to stimulate digestion and also to relieve stomach cramps and discomfort. Chamomile is known to calm the nerves, and this ancient herb's gentle yet effective nature makes it popular for use with children. Chamomile is historically known as a "does it all" type of herb: In traditional and historical herbal medicine, chamomile tends to its patients as an anti-inflammatory, a sedative, an antispasmodic, and more. Chamomile is celebrated for its soothing effects.

How to Use: Tea, tincture, infusion, bath soak, salve

Lore: The ancient Egyptians held the chamomile flower in high regard, using the crushed petals as part of their beautifying regimens. They dedicated the herb to their sun god, Ra, and believed it brought luck and prosperity. It was also used in the mummification process, as it covered the scent of decay. A natural healer, chamomile's presence in the garden is believed to assist nearby plants by encouraging them to thrive.

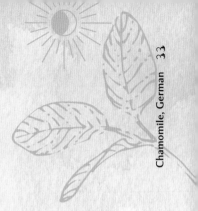

Magickal Uses: Chamomile is an herb to keep close. When planting around your house, include chamomile nearby to ward off negative energies. Chamomile has also been used in abundance spells and to attract money. In the springtime, chamomile is excellent for creating flower crowns to wear for Ostara and Beltane, and to honor the turning of the wheel of the year. Dried chamomile can be added to herbal bundles to burn in the home during purification rituals.

Easy Rituals, Potions, and Recipes: Chamomile is a beautiful addition to any nighttime tea. Blend with skullcap, lavender, and passionflower for a calming before-bed nightcap. Alternatively, create a chamomile tincture with apple cider vinegar or a spirit of your choice, and add a few drops to a tea of your choosing. To harness the purifying qualities of the flower, crush using a mortar and pestle, sprinkle the crushed flowers on any incense, and burn in your home or other sacred space.

CHICKWEED

Stellaria media

Star Weed

Chickweed is a low-growing, succulent plant, which some people consider a weed. It has delicate, small, white star-shaped flowers. Native to Europe and Asia, chickweed grows around the globe and is as comfortable in rural areas as it is in urban.

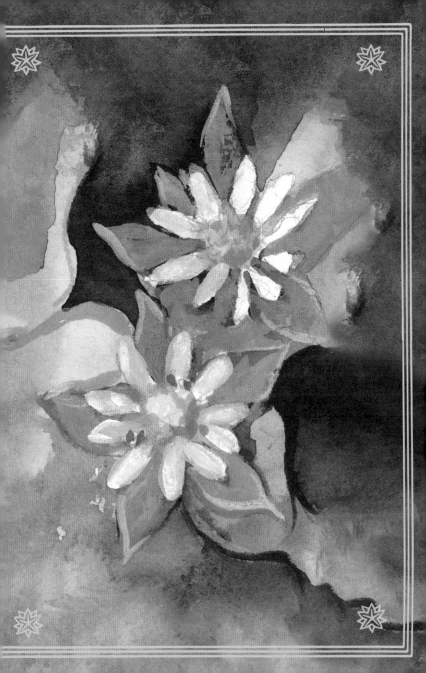

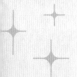

Parts Used: Leaves, flowers

Historical Medicinal Uses: Traditionally, chickweed was used in herbal medicine to encourage weight loss when ingested, and externally as a way to soothe skin irritations, especially itches. It's an incredibly gentle and supportive herbal ally and can be called upon as a tonic herb to support overall health and vitality.

How to Use: Infusion, tincture, powder, capsule, topical

Lore: European folklore holds that carrying a sprig of chickweed in a pocket can draw the attention of a loved one or ensure that a lover is faithful.

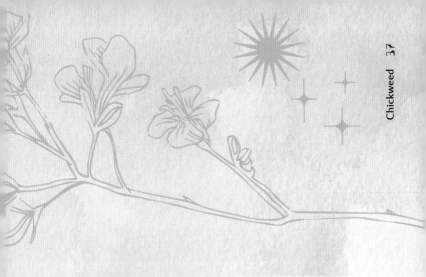

Magickal Uses: Chickweed is magickally associated with fidelity and love, and also connected to the moon. Much like the tides themselves, which are governed by the moon, chickweed honors the cycles and softness of all things. Known as a soothing herb, chickweed is ideal to connect with when you need to imbue the moment with a little sparkle from her starry blossoms.

Easy Rituals, Potions, and Recipes: Make a chickweed oil for skin support or for rituals of love drawing. Fill a mason jar with chickweed. Make sure it's been dried at least a few days, so that no water can get into your oil (that would spoil it). Cover with your favorite oil—olive and sunflower are both great. Poke it with chopsticks or a clean utensil to remove all air bubbles, and then cap. Set it on a plate and let it rest. Add more oil over the next few days if necessary. After six weeks, strain and use.

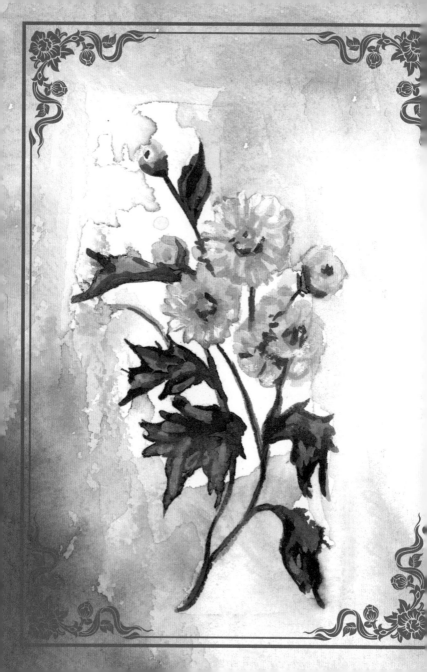

CHRYSANTHEMUM

Chrysanthemum x morifolium

Garden Mum

There are countless varieties of the beautiful blossoming chrysanthemum. Standing about 1 foot (30 cm) to 3 feet (1 m) high and almost as wide, the chrysanthemum's leaves are alternate and divided into leaflets with teeth, or sometimes smooth edges. They bloom in fall, and flowers display a lot of variety—sometimes a single flower and sometimes many—in a great myriad of colors.

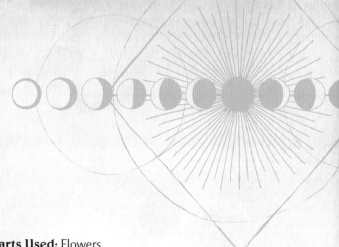

Parts Used: Flowers

Historical Medicinal Uses: Chrysanthemums were cultivated first in China as far back as 1500 BCE. In traditional Chinese medicine, chrysanthemums are a yin tonic that clears heat, acts as a blood purifier, and is considered deeply soothing and rejuvenating. During the Song dynasty, a cup of chrysanthemum tea was commonly taken to enjoy its benefits.

How to Use: Tincture, tea

Lore: In Chinese culture, the chrysanthemum was one of four noble plants, and a symbol of vitality. The ancient Greeks believed that wearing a garland of chrysanthemums would keep away evil spirits.

Magickal Uses: Chrysanthemums bloom in their many colors during Samhain season, when the veil between this world and the next grows thin, allowing messages from guides, spirits, and ancestors to come through. Samhain is usually celebrated from October 31 to November 1. During this time, hang a chrysanthemum wreath on your door to say hello to benevolent spirits, and to ward off unwanted presences.

Easy Rituals, Potions, and Recipes: All of the different colors of chrysanthemums make it ideal for practicing color magick. Go to your local flower shop and select, with an intention, a color of chrysanthemum you like for your home. Each day as you see the colored flower, work toward the intention that the color is helping you cultivate in your home. For example, red may resonate with passion, orange with perseverance, or yellow with creativity!

CLARY SAGE

Salvia sclarea

Eye Bright

A member of the mint family, clary sage is a biennial plant that stands approximately 3-4 feet (1-1.2 m) in height. The square stems are covered with thin hairs, and they are adorned with large purple, white, or pink flowers.

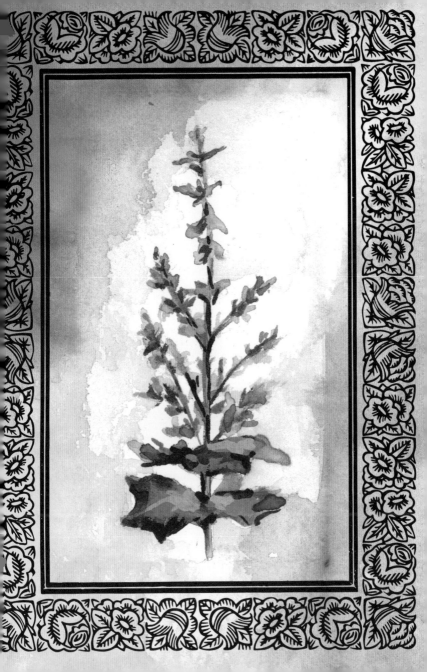

Parts Used: Flowering tops, leaves

Historical Medicinal Uses: The name *clary sage* comes from the Latin word "*claris*," or "clear." Not surprisingly, clary sage was traditionally used as a treatment for eye troubles. It was also called see bright, eye bright, and *oculus christi*.

How to Use: Essential oil

Lore: In ancient Rome, clary sage was used for a variety of ailments, including as an eyewash and to support the menstrual cycle. The seventeenth century, English herbalist Nicholas Culpeper warned of mixing wine with sage because of its intense effects as an aphrodisiac. Its aroma was said to reduce stress.

Magickal Uses: Clary sage is said to be both an intuition booster and an aphrodisiac. It knows the way between the worlds, and can be a potent guide for a dream-seeking traveler. Work with clary sage as you explore the depths.

Easy Rituals, Potions, and Recipes: An essential oil of clary sage can be an aid in your divination practice. Before reading tarot or oracle cards, calling on a pendulum, or scrying, put a small amount of oil on your third eye and ask clary sage for support.

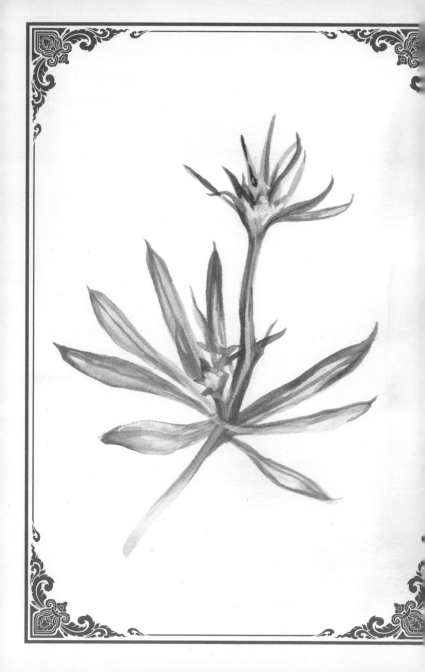

CLEAVERS

Galium aparine

The Red Root

Also known as bedstraw, cleavers seem to creep across the ground of the forest floor, thickets, and near the sea, growing low to the ground. It often covers other plants, attaching with their small, hooked hairs that grow out of the leaves and stems, earning the name "catchweed." It produces flowers with star-shaped petals that can be white to greenish in color.

Parts Used: Whole plant

Historical Medicinal Uses: Historically, the aerial parts of the plant (leaves and flowers) were made into a poultice or salve to treat bug bites, cuts, and other minor skin irritations. Modern-day herbalists may use cleavers as a diuretic when taken internally. Cleavers "get things moving," and because of this, it is used to clear stagnation and create more flow in the body. It is also a known substitute for coffee.

How to Use: Tea, tincture, poultice, salve, juice, tonic

Lore: Cleaver roots have been said to turn the bones red, probably because birds that ate the roots were seen to have red bones, and the roots yield a red dye. Because of the plant's hairlike and sticky constitution, it was historically used as stuffing for mattresses. Lore holds that if you throw cleavers against someone's back and they stick, that person has a lover or someone who would like to play that part; if the cleavers fall to the ground, they will form the first letter of the name of a lover who should appear shortly.

Magickal Uses: Cleavers are the very embodiment of tenacity. Whenever you're dealing with something that you find challenging to stick with, or when you're having trouble staying the course or just feel a bit defeated, cleaver magick may be just what you need.

Easy Rituals, Potions, and Recipes: Cleavers can be used in any spell that is intended for bringing things together. Place a pinch of cleavers into a small sachet, along with items representing the things you wish to bring together. Close the sachet and hold it in your hands. Sit quietly and meditate with the sachet, imagining the coming together of the things within. When you are finished, place the sachet on your altar for a full moon cycle.

COMFREY

Symphytum officinale

The Battlefield Herb

Comfrey is a large-leafed plant with hairy stems and oblong-shaped leaves. This plant grows in a busy fashion, up to 3 feet (1 m) high, and produces purple bell-shaped, five-lobed flowers. Comfrey can be found in the moist grasslands of Asia, Europe, and North America. This plant has fine hairs on both its stems and leaves, and its flowers can be white, pink, or purple.

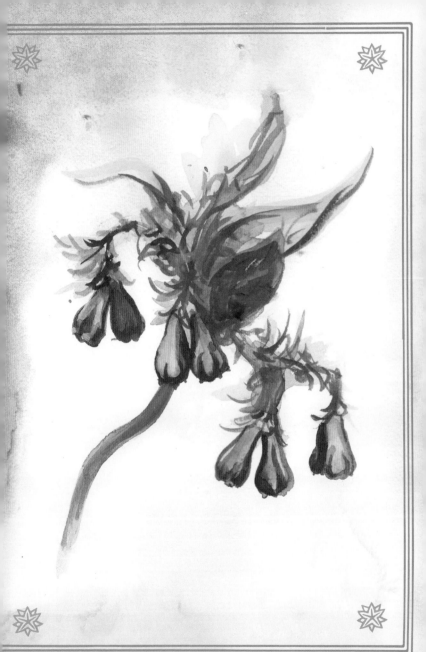

Parts Used: Leaves, root

Historical Medicinal Uses: Documented as a healing herb for thousands of years (mentioned by ancient Greek healer Pliny the Elder, among others), comfrey is known to have been cultivated since at least 400 BCE. It was used as an external aid in healing broken bones and to slow bleeding. It is also known for treating boils, abscesses, sprains, and bruises. Tea was taken to treat internal bleeding, diarrhea, ulcers, and other stomach issues. However, it is important to note that there has been much discussion of toxicity with comfrey for internal use in modern herbalism, and it should not be ingested.

How to Use: Tincture, poultice, salve, infusion (external use only)

Lore: Known as the "battlefield herb," comfrey was a staple in the bags of many battlefield medics during historical wars. Heated with water to create a poultice, and then applied with a bandage, the remedy would dry stiff and constrict the movement of broken and reset bones. The scientific name *Symphytum* comes from the Greek words meaning "grow together" and "plant." The common name, *comfrey*, comes from Latin, also meaning "to grow together."

Magickal Uses: Comfrey has been used traditionally in magickal practices to promote safe travels. Put a bit in your suitcase or carry it with you (as long as it's safe to travel with plants where you're headed) to ensure security while traveling. For a simple travel amulet, add a sprinkle of comfrey to a locket and wear it around your neck. An herb known for its ability to "join together," it makes a beautiful addition to love charms and abundance spells and can be added to jars and sachets. Place photos or representations of the two energies you wish to bring together into a jar or sachet, and sprinkle with comfrey while speaking your spell.

Easy Rituals, Potions, and Recipes: To create a poultice, simply crush the dried leaves and add a bit of water to make a "mush" or paste. Spread it on a sore area of the body, topped with gauze. (Be careful not to use comfrey on broken skin.) To create a lotion or muscle rub, infuse the herbs into a carrier oil, such as sweet almond. Let the oil and herb blend sit in a dark cabinet for a full moon cycle. Strain the spent herbs, thanking them for their medicine, and place them back into the earth. The oil can be used as is at that stage, or added to cocoa or shea butters to create a body butter or lotion.

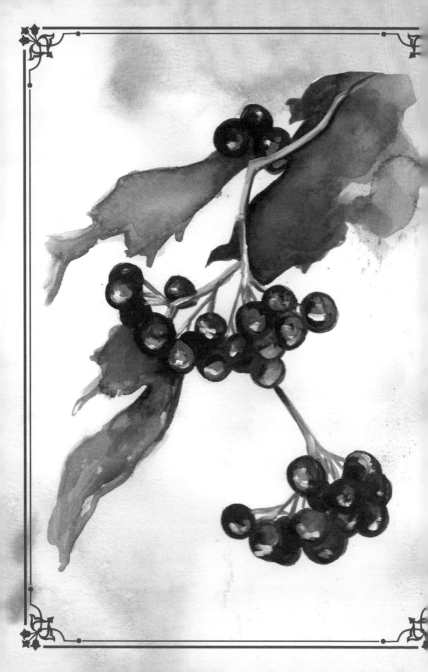

CRAMPBARK

Viburnum opulus

The Muscle Relaxer

Crampbark is an upright shrub, growing up to 16 feet (5 m) tall, with three-lobed, long, broad leaves. White corymb flowers grow at the tops of the stems with an outer ring of larger flowers. The plant produces small red berries.

Parts Used: Bark

Historical Medicinal Uses: True to its name, this herb has been traditionally used to ease abdominal cramps and relax muscles, especially those of the uterus, making it a popular herb to use during pregnancy. It is also commonly known as guelder rose.

How to Use: Tea, tincture

Lore: Historically, crampbark was used in rituals to aid women with healing. In Ukraine, it is also known as kalyna, after a goddess in Slavic mythology who was present during the birth of the universe. Representations of this herb are common in Ukrainian folk art. In some North American Indigenous cultures, crampbark has also been used as a tobacco substitute.

Magickal Uses: Crampbark is an herb connected to the feminine and the deep power of the womb. Use it in spells and rituals related to healing ancestral trauma, connecting to the divine feminine, and relieving mother-related emotional distress.

Easy Rituals, Potions, and Recipes: Create a simple tea by blending crampbark, ginger root, cinnamon, and orange peel. Sip during a full moon and enjoy your connection to mother moon!

DAMIANA

Turnera diffusa

Old Woman's Broom

Damiana is a small shrub that grows in southern Texas, Central America, South America, and the Caribbean. Its fragrant yellow flowers bloom low to the ground.

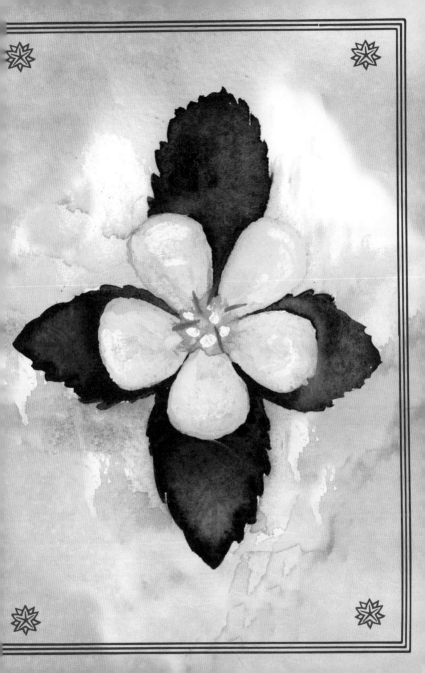

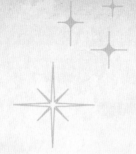

Parts Used: Leaves

Historical Medicinal Uses: Historically among the ancient Mayans, damiana was used as an aphrodisiac, said to increase desire. Damiana was also known as a wonderful herbal remedy to ease anxiety, nervousness, or depression, especially if those conditions were related to sexual issues. Some herbalists also used damiana to soothe digestive issues or as an elixir for overall wellness.

How to Use: Powder, tincture, tea

Lore: Folklore in Mexico claims that damiana was the key ingredient in the original margarita.

Magickal Uses: Because of its history as an aphrodisiac, damiana is a wonderful addition to any love spell, especially if it's related to sex magick. Keep some dried damiana in a sachet under your pillow or bed, or drink a damiana love spell tea to get into the mood.

Easy Rituals, Potions, and Recipes: Cast a love spell with damiana tea. Blend 1 teaspoon (5 g) each of dried damiana leaves, dried rose petals, and dried chamomile flowers. Let the blend steep in warm water, then strain or remove the tea ball or bag. Compost the herbs, asking the earth to hold you in love, and sip your tea while imagining an aura of love and support as damiana envelopes you in a sweet and tender embrace.

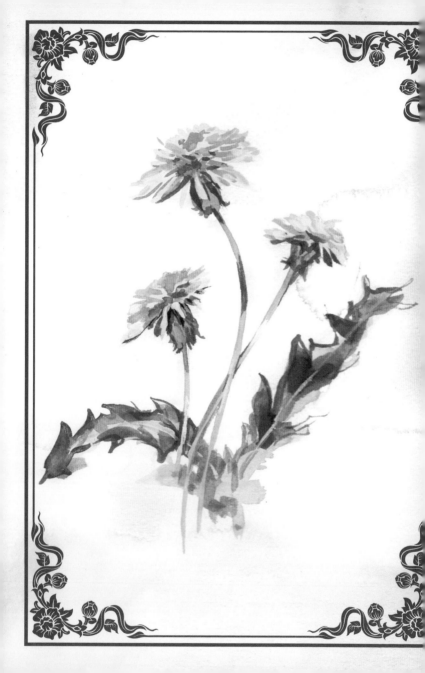

DANDELION

Taraxacum officinale

Tooth of the Lion

Ah, yes, the humble dandelion. The plant that everyone disregards as a common weed is actually packed full of nutrients. You'll know dandelion for its yellow blossoms that pop up across lawns and fields. Growing up to 18 inches (46 cm) tall, the thin stem produces one yellow flower with oblong petals and yellow florets. Basal, serrated leaves grow from the stem, which secretes a white milky latex when broken. (The name *dandelion* is believed to come from the French for "teeth of a lion," possibly due to the shape of the leaves.) Spent petals are replaced with wispy "balls" of seeds that blow away and produce new plants. (Make a wish!)

Parts Used: Whole plant

Historical Medicinal Uses: Historical uses of this herb are vast and varying, appearing in many cultures. Known as a diuretic, liver tonic, and diarrhea aid, it has been used to treat appendicitis and kidney disease. This versatile plant is currently being studied for its potential anticancer agents. Dandelions were historically used in medicine as a support to the digestive system, the urinary system, and the pancreas. Dandelion wine is also a lovely tonic.

How to Use: Tea, tincture, ingestion, infusion, decoction; bath blend, culinary uses

Lore: Dandelion is believed to have magickal properties that aid in the calling of spirits. Historical rituals incorporating dandelion were thought to increase psychic abilities and bring brightness and joy to one's life. In some folklore, the dandelion is associated with transformation. If you have a bad habit that you wish to move into the winds of change, set your intention before blowing on a gone-to-seed dandelion, and then watch the seeds (like your habit!) float away.

Magickal Uses: These yellow flowers can teach us about resilience and courage. Incorporate them into rituals for perseverance, inner strength, and buoyancy. With their sunny disposition, dandelions are always good for brightening up a place or situation. In mythology, dandelions have been associated with goddesses Aphrodite and Hecate.

Easy Rituals, Potions, and Recipes: If your garden or yard is like many others during the warmer months, it likely has dandelions sprouting up everywhere. Aside from being magickal wish makers, the leaves and roots of this "weed" make a delicious addition to your summer salads. Simply pull the plant from the ground with the root intact, thanking it for sharing its medicine. Cut the greens off at the base of the plant and wash both leaves and roots. Lay the roots flat on a baking sheet and roast in the oven at 350 degrees F for 15 to 20 minutes. Let them cool, chop into bite-sized pieces, and then add to your dish. You can also use dandelion in an herbal smoke bundle or use the petals in a tea or floral bath blend. Simply hang the greens and florets upside down to dry before adding.

ECHINACEA

Echinacea purpurea

The Cure-All

Echinacea grows up to 4 feet (1.2 m) in height with hairy leaves. Unbranched stems sprout purple flowers with oblong petals that grow slightly downward from the bristly center. A member of the daisy family, it flourishes naturally in Central and Eastern North America, but it is cultivated widely. Commonly known as purple coneflower.

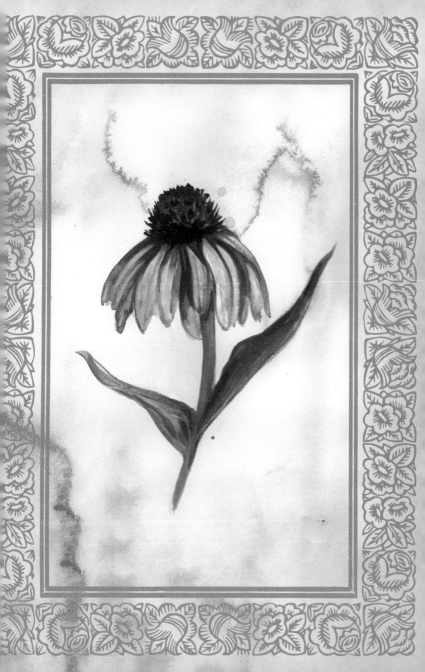

Parts Used: Roots, flower heads, leaves

Historical Medicinal Uses: Marketed in the 1800s as a blood thinner, echinacea was also used to treat snake bites, toothaches, burns, ulcers, coughs, and sore throats, so it is not surprising that it was known as "the cure-all" in many herbal traditions. Echinacea is a cooling and drying herb that has also traditionally been used as an immune strengthener. It is believed that this herb clears and tends to the lymph system and can help the body fight infections.

How to Use: Tea, tincture, poultice, juice

Lore: A popular herb used by many healers, echinacea is believed to bring strength and protection when carried, making it a popular addition to talismans and sachets. Legend has it that echinacea is associated with goddesses of the river. If you live near a river, offer a little echinacea as a gift.

Magickal Uses: Because of its history of immune strengthening and support, it's no surprise that the energy of echinacea is supportive as well. Carry a bit of echinacea with you to encourage resilience and success during trying times.

Easy Rituals, Potions, and Recipes: Dry echinacea by hanging it upside down from the stems. Once dry, pluck the leaves and petals and place them into a container, such as a tin or jar. Store it in your herbal medicine cabinet for use as a poultice for skin irritations such as bug bites, mild burns, scrapes, or rashes. When needed, remove the desired amount of herb from the container and add a bit of water. Mix until it forms a paste or mush and apply it to the desired area.

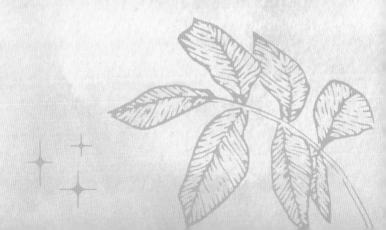

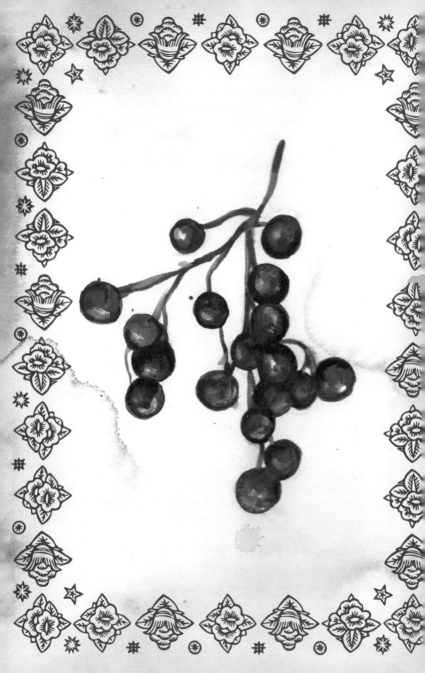

ELDER

Sambucus nigra

The Medicine Chest

Elder trees can be found naturally in a variety of conditions in Britain and Northern Europe but are cultivated widely. Trees grow 10-30 feet (3-9 m) tall, sprouting oblong leaflets growing opposite each other. White flowers grow in flat pinnacles. Fruit-bearing trees produce dark purple or black berries.

Parts Used: Flower, berries

Historical Medicinal Uses: Herbalists have long worked with elder in traditional medicine. Elder leaves were historically used to treat cuts, scrapes, sores, and abrasions, while the berries provided immune support at the onset of a cold or the flu. Elder remains a popular staple herb in many modern herbalists' remedies.

How to Use: Tea, tincture, syrup, decoction

Lore: Elder trees were sacred to the Celtic peoples of old; it is said that a wise-woman nymph named Elda Mor resides in the elder tree, watching over it and those who harvest it for healing. Planted near a home, it is believed to ward off evil spirits and provide protection. In some mythologies, it is said that mischievous spirits live within the elder. To properly harvest it, permission must be granted, and all gathering must be done with respect (as with all plants!).

Magickal Uses: Like its name, this tree carries deep, old wisdom. Call on the magick of the elder to support you in rituals and spells for protection and boundary-setting. Elder can also be used in cord-cutting rituals. Sprinkle in front of the thresholds of your home to protect it from negative energy.

Easy Rituals, Potions, and Recipes: Elderberries have antioxidant properties. Create an elderberry syrup to take as a daily tonic for immune support: Fill a small pot with 3 cups (690 ml) of water, and add ½ half cup (112 g) of elderberries. (Add ginger root, cinnamon, and cloves for extra flavor!) Bring the mixture to a boil and cook for approximately 5 minutes. Turn off the heat and allow to steep for at least 30 minutes. When it has reached room temperature, pour the mixture through a double layer of cheesecloth into a pourable container. Squeeze all the liquid out of the herbs and thank them for their medicine. Add honey and stir until completely dissolved. Pour the liquid into a small clean bottle with a lid. Label and store in the fridge.

ELECAMPANE

Inula helenium

Horse heal

Elecampane, also known as horse heal or elf dock, is an herb that is often considered a weed, originating in Europe and northern Asia, but naturalized in eastern North America where is grows easily along roadsides and in fields. Elecampane grows from 4-8 feet (1.2-2.4 m) tall, with toothed, hairy leaves and yellow flowers that resemble sunflowers.

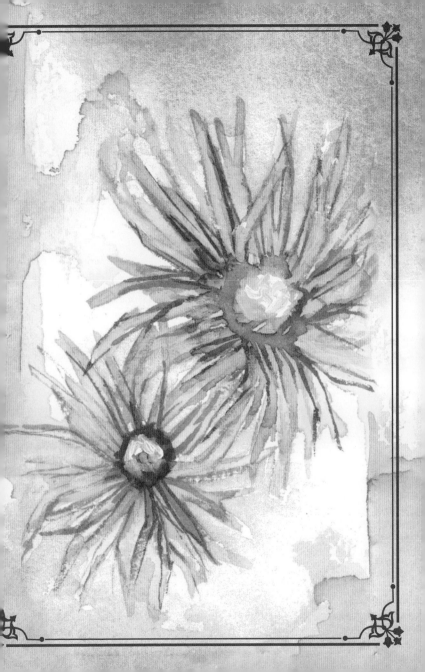

Parts Used: Root, leaves

Historical Medicinal Uses: This herb has been used in traditional medicine since the ancient Greeks and Romans. Pliny the Elder noted that the Emperor Augustus's daughter took a cheering tonic of elecampane daily. Elecampane was known as a clearing herb, good for moving phlegm out of the body. It was also considered to be useful as a respiratory support—including for horses—and historically was used to treat coughs.

How to Use: Powder, tincture, glycerite, wash

Lore: Elecampane's scientific name, *helenium*, comes from the story of Helen of Troy. It was believed that where her tears fell, elecampane blossomed.

Magickal Uses: This herb has been used magickally to clear stagnation, banish, protect, and support in rituals and spells. Ritually, elecampane can be called upon in a variety of ways. You may want to meditate a bit with the plant and see what its spirit whispers to you.

Easy Rituals, Potions, and Recipes: Elecampane is known for its powerful work in protection magick and banishing spells. Crush a bit of dried elecampane into a floor wash to help clear stagnant energy and to envelop your home in supportive protection. While there are a variety of ways to craft a floor wash, depending on what surface your floor is and what you have on hand, consider mixing the herbs with hot water in a French press or creating a tea, straining the herbs, and then adding a bit of white vinegar.

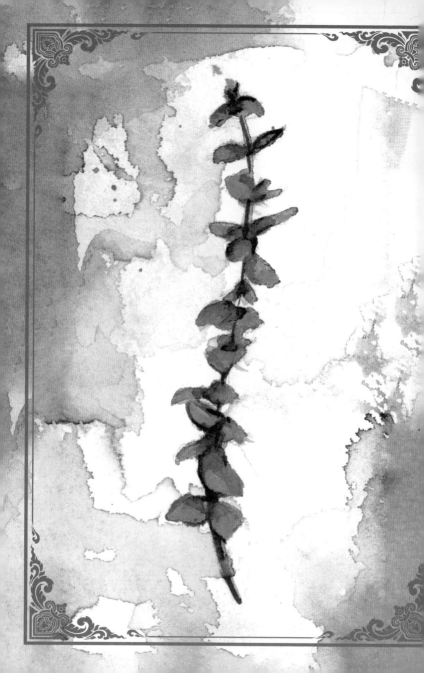

EUCALYPTUS

Eucalyptus globulus

Fever Tree

The eucalyptus is a tall, aromatic evergreen tree native to Australia (where it is often called gum tree), but it is grown widely around the world. Eucalyptus trees have a distinctive papery bark. Their leaves are a dark, glossy green, and, like other plants in the myrtle family, they are covered in oil glands, which produce a precious essential oil.

Parts Used: Leaves, twigs

Historical Medicinal Uses: Eucalyptus oil has long been used in traditional medicine. Historically, its oil was used to treat respiratory struggles, including easing congestion. It was also considered helpful for topical wounds. In traditional Aboriginal medicine, eucalyptus was employed to treat fevers. Ritual bathing practices using eucalyptus have been documented in many cultures, including Nordic and Japanese.

How to Use: Infusion, tincture, essential oil

Lore: For the Indigenous peoples of Australia, the eucalyptus tree is sacred; it symbolizes the division between the underworld, earth, and heaven.

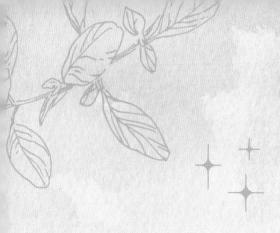

Magickal Uses: Representing purity, leaves from a eucalyptus plant can be burned, added to a bath, or crafted into salves as part of a ritual or magickal practice. Hang the leaves and branches over a bed or tuck them into pillowcases as a gentle plant ally.

Easy Rituals, Potions, and Recipes: To enjoy its distinctive and delightful scent, hang a eucalyptus branch in your shower or tip a few drops of oil into your bath. A wonderful way to work with eucalyptus and water is through ritual bathing. A ritual bath is one drawn and performed to ritually cleanse, purify, relax, and connect with the self (you can craft an intention for a bath around anything relevant in your daily life, as water is incredibly healing). To do this, add eucalyptus leaves to a piece of cheesecloth, tie it up into a sachet, drop it into the bath, and let it sit for a few minutes before you enter the water. As the water drains at the end of the bath, imagine all the energy that is not yours traveling with the water down the drain.

FENNEL

Foeniculum vulgare

Greek Sacred Herb

Fennel can grow up to 5 feet (1.5 m) tall, with light, feathery foliage. It bears yellow, flat umbels, each with 20 to 50 tiny yellow flowers; seeds are small and oval. Fennel is a sweet-smelling herb. Though its roots are in the Mediterranean, it is grown globally.

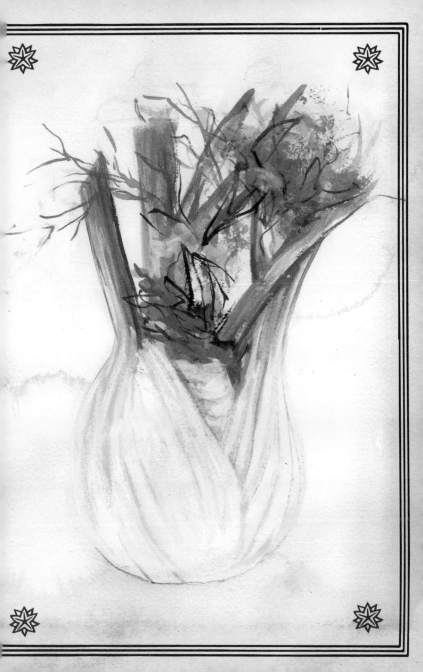

Parts Used: Seeds, bulb, leaves

Historical Medicinal Uses: Fennel has been historically used as a digestive aid; it was known as a reliever of stomach cramps, indigestion, heartburn, and bloating. Fennel is also an essential kitchen herb dating at least as far back as the ancient Greeks. It is also one of the primary components of the spirit absinthe.

How to Use: Tea, tincture, decoction; culinary uses

Lore: The ancient Roman herbalist Pliny the Elder wrote that snakes would eat fennel to improve their eyesight after they shed their skins. His belief that fennel was an especially powerful healing herb carried through centuries and cultures. In the Middle Ages, the peoples of the British Isles hung fennel from door frames on Midsummer's Eve to ward off evil spirits. In medieval Italy, witches may have fought late-night battles using fennel stalks as their weapons against rival covens. Fennel is popular in Ayurvedic treatments as well.

Magickal Uses: In magickal practices, you can work with the entire fennel plant or just its seeds. Grown it near your doors as a protective plant or place fennel seeds around your home to cast out negative energies.

Easy Rituals, Potions, and Recipes: Fennel is a kitchen witch's dream herb. While baking or preparing a meal, sprinkle fennel into your recipe while whispering your intent. Envision the intent being infused into the meal along with the fennel.

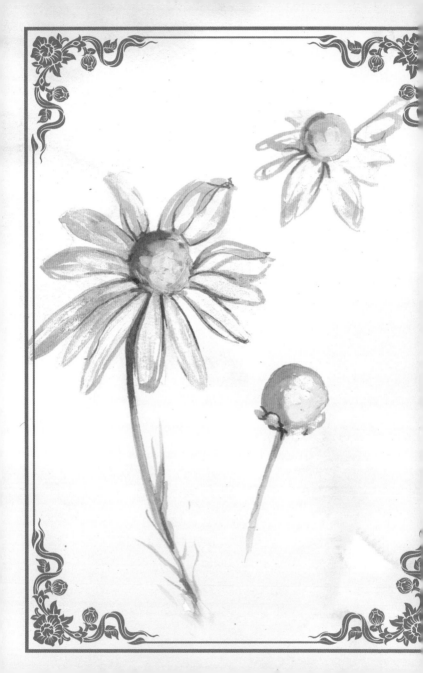

FEVERFEW

Tanacetum parthenium

The Devil's Daisy

A small, bushy plant with diminutive ray-shaped flowers, similar to daisies. Alternate, yellowish-green hairy leaves give off a bitter odor when crushed.

Parts Used: Leaves, root, seeds

Historical Medicinal Uses: Feverfew was used in ancient times by Egyptians and Greeks to cure general aches and pains as well as to ease menstrual cramps. More recently, it is known as a natural aid for relieving migraines, nausea, and respiratory ailments such as coughs.

How to Use: Decoction, tincture

Lore: During the plague in Medieval Europe, feverfew was planted near homes in the belief that it would keep occupants safe from the disease. It is possible that such efforts could have proven somewhat effective because feverfew contains the chemical pyrethrin, which is a known pest repellent, and may have kept out mice and rats that were infected with the disease.

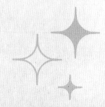

Magickal Uses: Feverfew is helpful in breaking curses and can be used to cut any cords of negative energy that have attached to you or your home. Additionally, placing the leaves of feverfew into a sachet that you carry with you is a magickal way to prevent accidents while traveling or out and about.

Easy Rituals, Potions, and Recipes: Place some feverfew flowers in a vase near the entry to your home to create a beautiful aesthetic while secretly establishing a barrier of protection from negative energy.

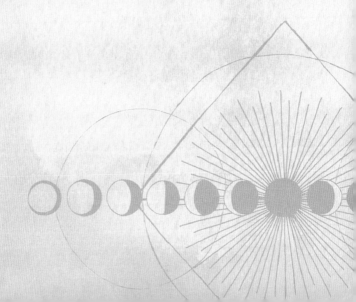

GINGER

Zingiber officinale

---

*The Expecting
Mother's Herb*

Ginger's reedlike stems grow to an average of 3 feet (1 m) tall and produce elongated green leaves with a spiky, cone-shaped flower emerging from the top. Their thick rhizomes (the part you may be most familiar with in the kitchen) are dug up after the leaves die.

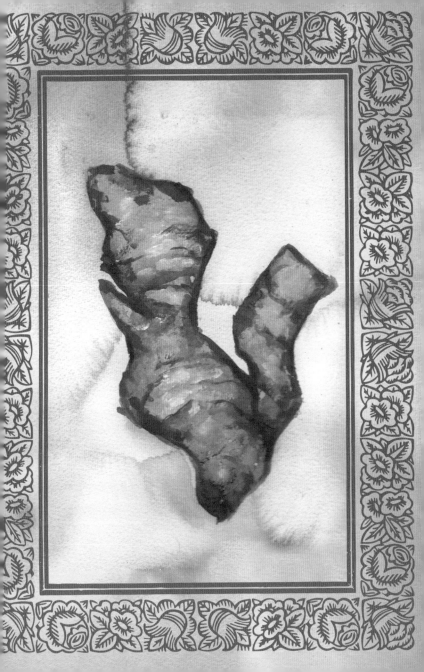

Parts Used: Rhizomes

Historical Medicinal Uses: Ginger root has been used to ease nausea and stomach ailments for centuries. Decocted and made into tea, it is a popular herb for use in early-term pregnancy to relieve the symptoms of morning sickness. Herbalists recommend ginger for all digestive system issues, as an anti-inflammatory ingredient, and for its antioxidant properties.

How to Use: Tea, tincture, decoction, ingestion, poultice, syrup, infusion

Lore: Long used in Asian cooking, ginger originated in India and southeast Asia and made its way to Europe with traders; it had become a popular ingredient in baked goods by the sixteenth century. Legend states that Queen Elizabeth I of England ordered biscuits to be baked in the shape of favored courtiers, which may be the origin of the whimsical "gingerbread people" cookies.

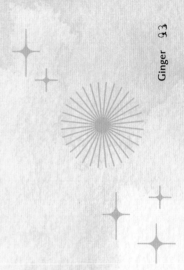

Magickal Uses: Ginger is believed to add "fire" to love spells, making them potent while accelerating the process. Given ginger's warming properties, be sure to incorporate it into spells, rituals, or gatherings where a little heat is called for! This may be in spellwork as an accelerator, when you're a little anxious, or when working with love magick. It is said that those who plant ginger in their gardens will attract money and prosperity.

Easy Rituals, Potions, and Recipes: Blend a tea or tincture of ginger root, damiana leaf, and rose petals to create a warming sex or love magick potion. Enjoy with your partner or alone.

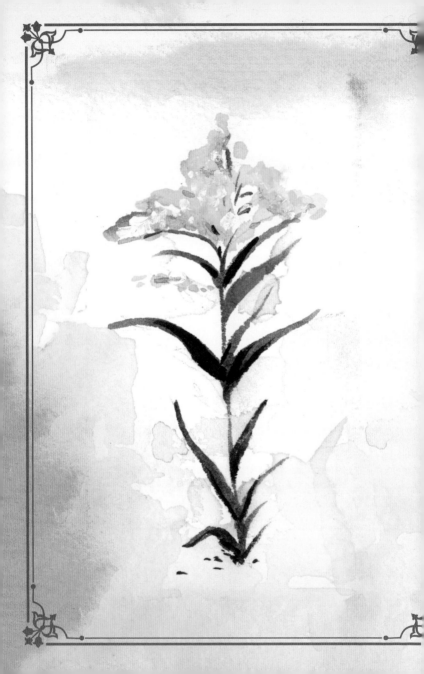

Goldenrod

Solidago virgaurea

Wound Weed

A tall herb with a simple stem that reaches 2-4 feet (0.6-1.2 m), goldenrod is considered by some to be a weed. Its yellow, late-blooming flowers appear near the top of the stem. Goldenrod grows widely in North America, and several species also grow in Asia and Europe.

Parts Used: Whole plant

Historical Medicinal Uses: The name *solidago* means "to make whole." Goldenrod has long been used in traditional healing both internally and externally. Internally, goldenrod was taken as a diuretic as well as to help counter allergy symptoms. Externally, salves made of goldenrod were used to treat wounds.

How to Use: Infusion, tincture, glycerite, salve

Lore: Legend has it that if goldenrod appears by your door unexpectedly, good fortune is headed your way. In United States history, it is said that "liberty tea" was brewed from goldenrod after the Boston Tea Party saw imported teas dumped into the harbor.

Magickal Uses: In magickal rituals and spell work, use goldenrod in love-drawing spells, as well as abundance spells. Add a bit of dried goldenrod to spell jars to support either of these intentions.

Easy Rituals, Potions, and Recipes: According to some folklore, goldenrod stems can be used as dowsing rods. The flower bobs when the user points the stems in the correct direction. Dowse with goldenrod to find lost objects or perhaps uncover an unexpected treasure. This is especially fun to do with any little witches in your life.

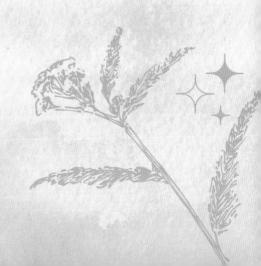

GOLDENSEAL

Hydrastis canadensis

Liquid Gold

Goldenseal is in the buttercup family and is native to eastern North America. It is a flowering plant with a single white flower that, when fertilized, grows into raspberry-like fruit. This striking woodland herb emerges from a yellow, knotted rootstock, producing a purplish hairy stem. The plant has hairy leaves and single, small, inconspicuous flowers; it blooms in the spring.

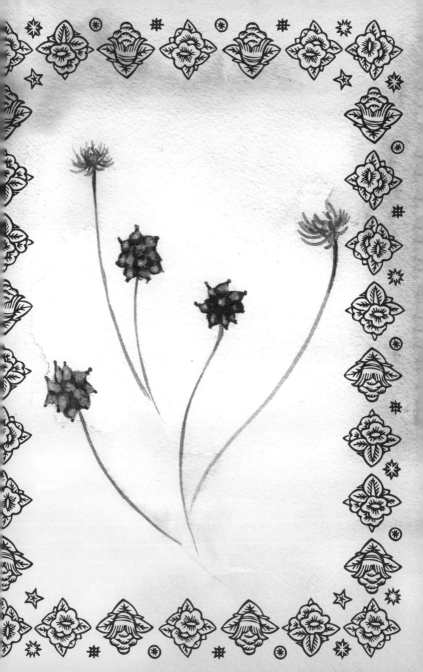

Parts Used: Root

Historical Medicinal Uses: This endangered plant was historically used as a digestive aid. A known bitter, it has been used traditionally as a remedy for hemorrhoids and bowel syndromes, as well as skin and eye washes. Additionally, the root produced a yellow stain that was used to dye clothing. Because of overharvesting, golden-seal is now endangered and should be treated with care.

How to Use: Tincture, salve, decoction, tea

Lore: Said to be bound to Venus and fire, goldenseal is believed to attract love and prosperity when sprinkled at the base of a golden candle. Because of its popularity in folk healing traditions, goldenseal has acquired a long list of common names, including yellow root, ground raspberry, yellow puccoon, wild circuma, eye-root, eye-balm, yellow paint, wild turmeric, and yelloweye.

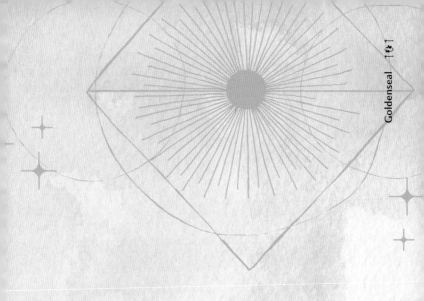

Magickal Uses: Calling on the energy of goldenseal is a good way to support a money-drawing spell; it is helpful in support of any ritual involving financial matters.

Easy Rituals, Potions, and Recipes: Create a prosperity pouch with goldenseal by sewing a golden pouch. You will need two small squares of gold or yellow fabric, green thread, a needle, a piece of paper, and some goldenseal. Sitting in ritual, write the words *abundance, prosperity*, and any others that feel appropriate on the piece of paper. Fold it small enough that it can fit into the pouch you are about to sew. With intent, sew three sides of the squares, creating a space for the folded paper and herbs. Place them into the pouch and sew the fourth side, closing them in. Place the pouch on your altar or sacred space as a talisman for attracting prosperity and financial security.

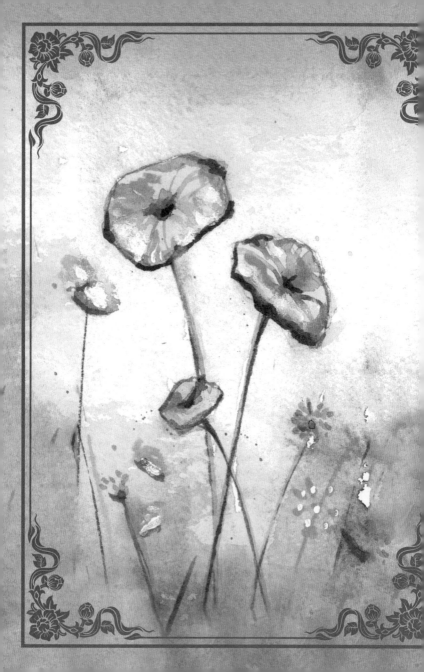

GOTU KOLA

Centella asiatica

Marsh Penny

A low, creeping plant that grows in swampy areas, gotu kola has fan-shaped green leaves and white or light-purple flowers. It yields a small oval-shaped fruit. Native to Southeast Asia, it thrives in tropical climates.

Parts Used: Leaves

Historical Medicinal Uses: Historically, gotu kola has been an herb celebrated in ancient Ayurvedic and Chinese medicine, particularly for use in supporting memory and brain function. It has also been used topically to treat wounds and skin conditions.

How to Use: Tincture, powder, infusion, capsule

Lore: Gotu kola has been called "the fountain of life," thanks to a Chinese folktale that told of an herbalist who lived for over two hundred years due to regular consumption of gotu kola. It was a favorite herb of monks for its ability to bring calmness and clarity to the mind.

Magickal Uses: In rituals and magickal practices, call on gotu kola when you need mental clarity or a tranquil mind.

Easy Rituals, Potions, and Recipes: Brew a gotu kola tea from fresh or dried leaves and add a touch of honey to prepare for meditation.

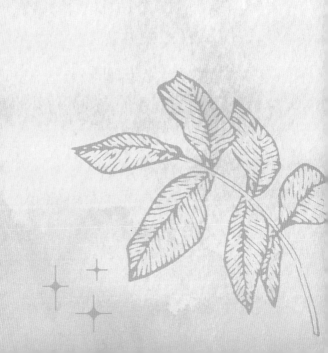

Gumweed

Grindelia spp.

The Sticky Herb

Gumweed is a bushy plant with sticky, rough stems; it can grow singly or in groups. Oblong leaves and yellow daisy-like flowers have overwrapping ray-shaped petals with a yellow center. Gumweed plants emit a milky sap or resin. It belongs to a group of plants in the aster family and is native to the Americas.

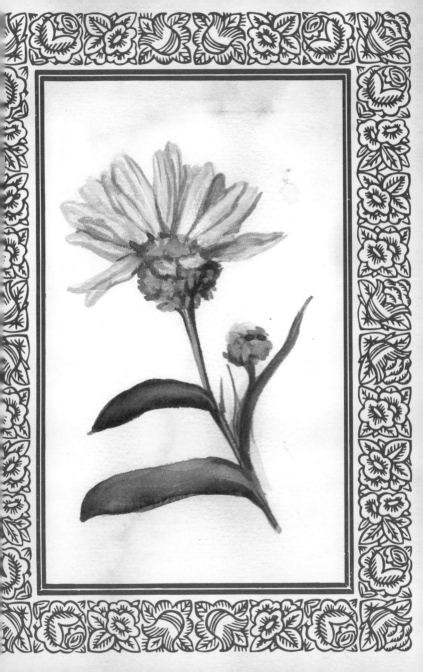

Parts Used: Aerial parts (all the parts above the soil)

Historical Medicinal Uses: Historically, gumweed has been used to treat respiratory ailments, and particularly as an expectorant for coughs and colds. Indigenous peoples of the Americas used gumweed as an effective remedy for topical skin irritations such as rashes, burns, bites, and poison ivy reactions.

How to Use: Tea, tincture, salve

Lore: True to its name, the resinous sap from this herb was an early example of chewing gum.

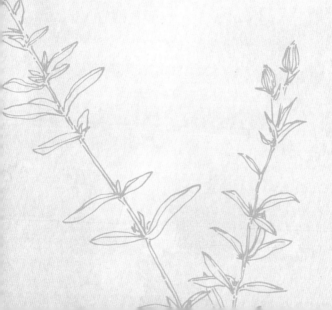

Magickal Uses: Gumweed's stickiness and ability to attract makes it an ideal herb to use in ritual. Gumweed is believed to aid in calling upon ancestor spirit guides to help locate an ailment in a person's body. Once the problem was located, gumweed or another herbal remedy could be used for treatment.

Easy Rituals, Potions, and Recipes: Burn the entire flower top of gumweed, or sprinkle small pieces into the flame of a purple candle when calling up ancestors and spirit guides.

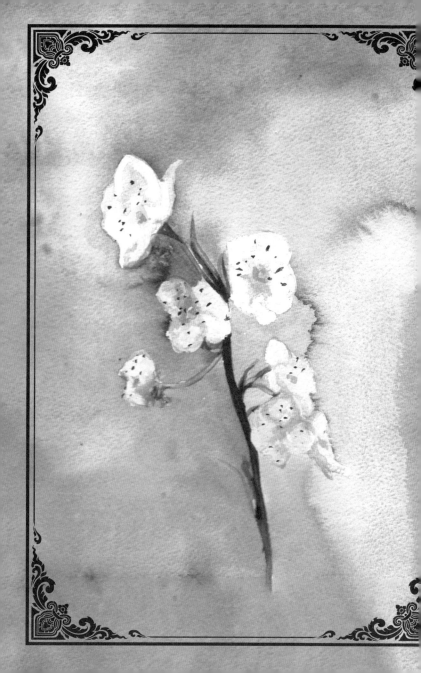

HAWTHORN

Crataegus oxyacantha

The Heart Herb

The hawthorn tree, also known as May tree, whitethorn, or haw berry, can be found in Europe, Asia, North Africa, and North America. It is a tall, thorny-branched tree with white blossoms and elliptic or oval-shaped leaves. The flowers transform into bright-red, berrylike pommes.

Parts Used: Berries, flowers, leaves

Historical Medicinal Uses: Starting with the ancient Romans, who used hawthorn as a tonic, this herb has been used medicinally throughout history. It is known for treating cardiovascular system problems and is also useful as a digestive aid and to combat insomnia.

How to Use: Tea, tincture, ingestion, decoction, syrup

Lore: Hawthorn has long been considered a symbol of love. In England, hawthorn trees were tied with ribbons during Beltane, and people would make wishes on the trees and ask for blessings from the deities and the divine. Maypoles were traditionally made from hawthorn, and crowns and wreaths of its blossoms are still prevalent during these springtime celebrations. In Welsh lore, hawthorn is associated with legend of the Lady of May, who scattered a trail of hawthorn petals that became the Milky Way. It is said that hawthorn branches and thorns were used in Jesus Christ's crown of thorns.

Magickal Uses: It is bad luck to disturb a hawthorn, and they should always be treated with the greatest respect. It's been said that if you tie ribbons around a hawthorn tree as a gift to the spirit of the tree and the Fae are nearby, you may be granted a wish. Use hawthorn in rituals of love and fertility and when working with the Fae.

Easy Rituals, Potions, and Recipes: Use hawthorn branches and flowers to create a Beltane flower crown. Simply weave them together (and feel free to add an array of other colorful flowers) to honor the Celtic turn of the wheel.

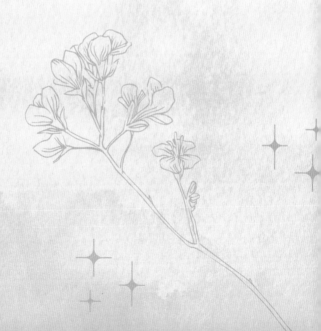

HIBISCUS

Hibiscus rosa-sinensis

Rose of China

Part of a large family of flowering plants, the hibiscus is known for its large red (or sometimes white, pink, blue, and more!) trumpet-shaped flowers.

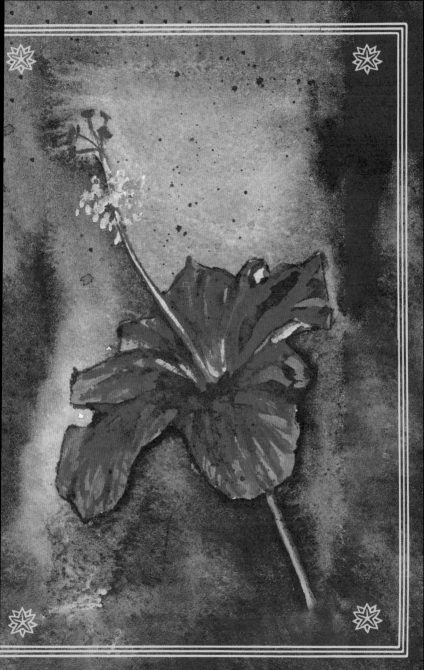

Parts Used: Flower

Historical Uses: Hibiscus is the national flower of Malaysia and has been used throughout Malay healing traditions. Hibiscus has been beloved for its ability to help with headaches, respiratory issues, and fever in traditional and historical herbal practices.

How to Use: Tea, topically

Lore: The hibiscus is also the state flower of Hawaii. Indigenous peoples in Hawaii would wear a hibiscus behind their ears to show relationship status. It is also seen as a welcoming symbol of friendship.

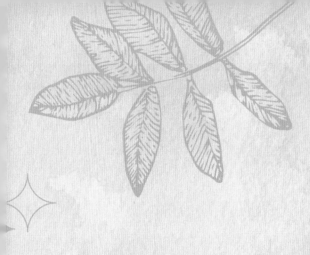

Magickal Uses: Associated with passion, hibiscus can be a potent addition to love spells.

Easy Rituals, Potions, and Recipes: Known in Mexico as Agua de Jamaica, this version of iced tea is refreshing and delicious. Heat four cups (920 ml) of water in a medium saucepan, adding ½ cup to 1 cup (100-200 g) of sugar (depending on how sweet you want this beverage). Add cinnamon, ginger slices, and a few allspice berries (optional). Heat the mixture until it boils and the sugar has dissolved. Add 1 cup (225 g) of hibiscus flowers (dried or fresh) and allow the drink to steep for twenty minutes before straining, chilling, adding water to the concentrate, and serving. Add a lime as a garnish for a little added citrus touch.

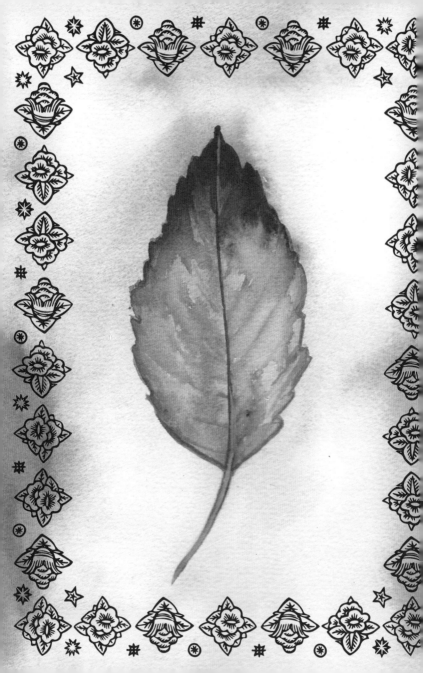

HOLY BASIL

Ocimum sanctum

Queen of the Herbs

A shrubby plant that grows 3 feet (1 m) high, holy basil has green or purple leaves that grow in opposites. The stem is slightly hairy, topped with small white or purple flowers. Holy basil is an aromatic plant and member of the mint family. Native to Southeast Asia, it is now cultivated widely. (Note that this is a different plant from sweet basil, _Ocimum basilicum._)

Parts Used: Leaves, flowering tops

Historical Medicinal Uses: Also known as tulsi, holy basil has a long history as a remedy for respiratory ailments, and is hailed as an effective decongestant and mucus thinner. It is specially celebrated in Ayurvedic medicine traditions. Historically, it has been used as an adaptogen (a substance that helps the body adapt to stress) and a tonic for overall well-being.

How to Use: Tea, tincture, infusion, poultice, essential oil

Lore: Holy basil is believed to have grown from the ground at the site where Jesus Christ was crucified, and is a symbol of holiness in the Greek Orthodox religion. In Hindu culture, holy basil is considered a reincarnation of Lakshmi, goddess of abundance, love, and beauty, and is therefore known for its divinity.

Magickal Uses: Holy basil is known as "the great protector." Work with it in rituals for protection, or cultivate it near or within your home as a protective plant.

Easy Rituals, Potions, and Recipes: Holy basil is beautiful and healing as an essential oil; it is believed to boost overall wellness, as well as respiratory health, when inhaled. Put a few drops into your favorite diffuser to cleanse and freshen the air in your home.

Hyssop

Hyssopus officinalis

Holy Herb

Hyssop is an evergreen shrub in the mint family. Native to the Middle East and southern Europe, hyssop is cultivated widely. It has narrow, dark-green leaves and beautiful, fragrant pink, purple, blue, and sometimes white flowers.

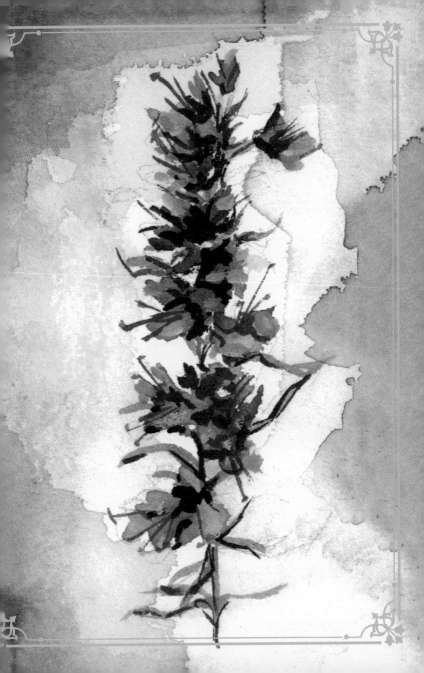

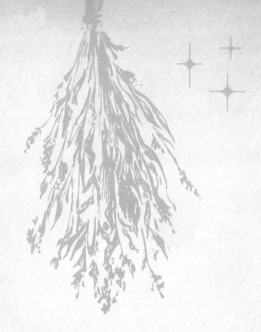

Parts Used: Aerial parts (all the parts above the soil)

Historical Medicinal Uses: Historically, hyssop has been used as a cure for respiratory ailments and is known for its cough suppressant qualities.

How to Use: Tea, tincture

Lore: In ancient Egypt, hyssop was used in rites of religious purification, and priests would consume hyssop with their bread. References to hyssop appear in ancient texts, including the Judeo-Christian bible.

Magickal Uses: Because of hyssop's historical association with purification, modern-day witches work with it for cleansing, purifying, and protection. If you're working to repel the evil eye or any kind of harmful energy, craft a charm or sachet with hyssop and carry it for protection.

Easy Rituals, Potions, and Recipes: A ritual bath is a wonderful way to receive the cleansing benefits of hyssop. Pack cheesecloth, a tea ball, or a bag with dried hyssop and allow it to soak in your bathwater (this makes for an easier cleanup; however, if you wish to let the plant float in the water, that works well too). As you bathe and then drain the water from the tub, focus on letting the hyssop water pull away any energies that don't belong to you. If you don't have a bathtub, get creative! A foot soak can be another beautiful way to work with this herb.

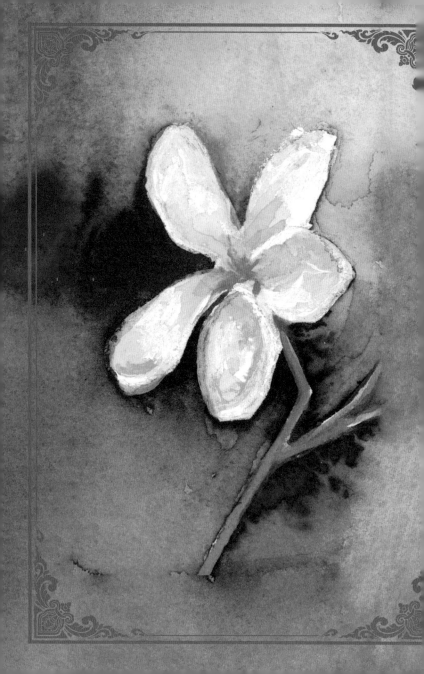

JASMINE

Jasminum sp.

Poet's Jasmine

There are over two hundred species of the flowering-shrub jasmine, which belongs to the olive family. Native to Asia, it has traveled widely and is cultivated and naturalized in many places. Jasmine is recognizable by starlike, incredibly fragrant flowers, often white or yellow.

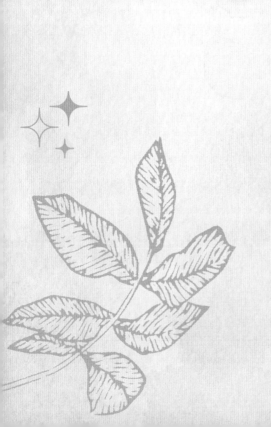

Parts Used: Flowers

Historical Medicinal Uses: Historically, jasmine has been considered an aphrodisiac and has long been beloved by perfumers for its strong, sweet scent. Renaissance physicians used jasmine in ointments for skin irritations and dry skin.

How to Use: Essential oil, incense

Lore: Because jasmine is an evening-blooming flower, it is associated with the moon and goddesses of the moon, and their female energy.

Magickal Uses: Jasmine can be included in spells for attracting love and prosperity. It can also be used to connect with the dreamworld and encourage prophetic dreams.

Easy Rituals, Potions, and Recipes: Make a dreaming sachet or pouch with dried jasmine blossoms when you want to listen to messages from the moon. Add additional magickal items such as amethyst, a written intention on a piece of parchment, or dried mugwort to the sachet.

JUNIPER BERRY

Juniperus spp.

Common Juniper

Junipers belong to the cypress family and are coniferous plants that may be shrubs or trees. They have needlelike leaves and brown, papery bark. The berries on a juniper are not true berries but more akin to cones that have a berrylike structure, starting out green and eventually ripening to blue-black or purple. They grow widely throughout the northern hemisphere.

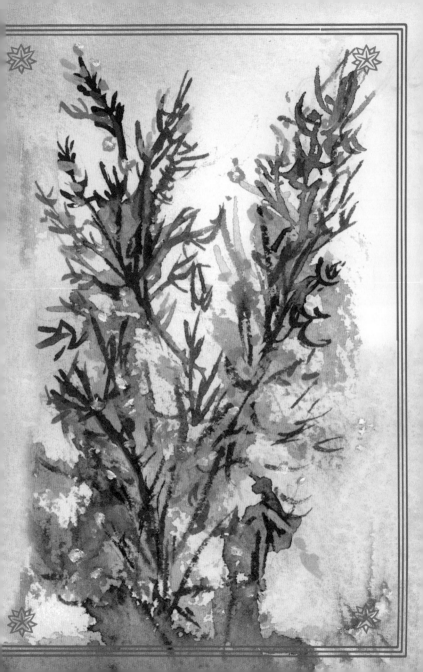

Parts Used: Berry

Historical Medicinal Uses: In traditional herbal medicine, juniper berry has been used in many cultures around the world for stomach troubles. Known for its stimulant and antiseptic properties, it was used by North American Indigenous peoples for respiratory troubles and kidney issues. Juniper essential oil has also long been used in aromatherapy. Juniper berries are what originally gave gin its distinctive flavor.

How to Use: Tincture, tea, essential oil, infusion

Lore: Juniper berries have been found in the tombs of ancient Egypt, where they were suggested as a cure for tapeworm. However, they were not traditionally grown there and may have been imported from Greece, where the ancient Greek physician Galen mentioned them as a cleanse for the liver and kidneys.

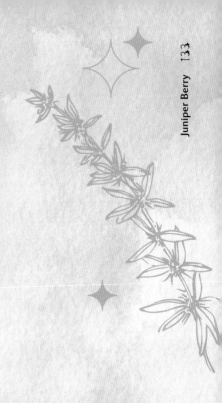

Magickal Uses: For modern green witches, juniper berries can be used in protection spells and rituals.

Easy Rituals, Potions, and Recipes: Make a juniper berry garland to hang in your home. This is a great ritual to do with little witches, especially during Winter Solstice and Yule time. Take a few boughs of juniper with berries on the branches and tie them with evergreen or holly. Hang them over a door for protection during the dark months.

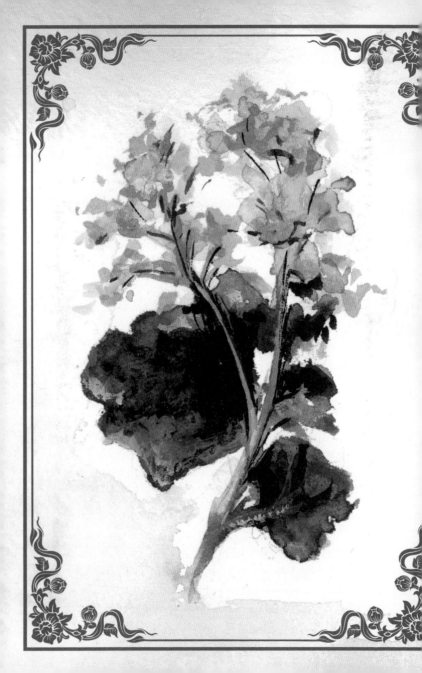

LADY'S MANTLE

Alchemilla vulgaris

Lion's Foot

A member of the rose family, lady's mantle is a perennial wildflower with distinctive round, scalloped leaves and tiny, yellow seasonal flowers. Lady's mantle is known for the way it collects dew in its leaves.

Parts Used: Leaves, flowers

Historical Medicinal Uses: Lady's mantle is known historically as a reproductive health herb. Herbalists would use it to treat heavy menstruation and cramps. The medieval herbalist Nicholas Culpeper found it useful to treat wounds.

How to Use: Infusion, tincture

Lore: Legend has it that during the Middle Ages, alchemists would collect the dew of lady's mantle and add it to their elixirs.

Magickal Uses: Include lady's mantle in releasing rituals or when crafting charms for fertility.

Easy Rituals, Potions, and Recipes: Taking a page from the alchemists and call upon lady's mantle when you wish to transform a part of your life. In the cycle of death and rebirth, letting go of what needs to die is an important step, making space for what is to come next. Sleep with lady's mantle under your pillow, or carry it as a charm to support you and hold you through this process.

LAVENDER

Lavandula officinalis

Queen of Plants

Lavender is a small evergreen shrub typically 1–2 feet (30–61 cm) in height, with grayish-green leaves; its long shoots are topped with purple flowers. A member of the mint family, lavender is native to the Mediterranean region but grown widely around the world.

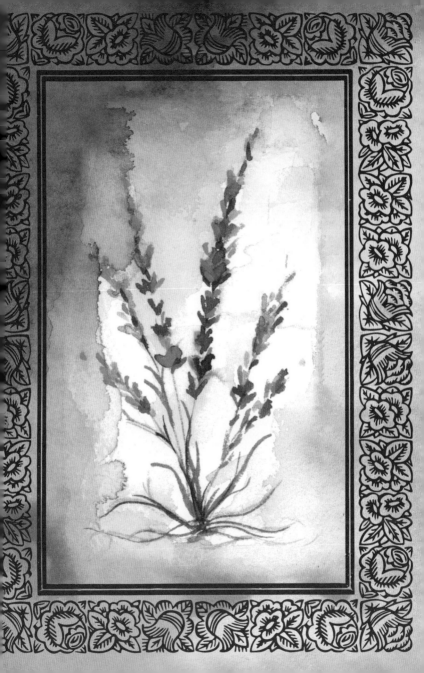

Parts Used: Flowers

Historical Medicinal Uses: One of herbalists' most popular plants since ancient times, lavender is well known as a soothing herb, used to ease tension and anxiety. It is also a sleep aid and inducer of sweet dreams. In the fourteenth century, King Charles of France was said to have required that his pillow be stuffed with lavender to ensure a good sleep.

How to Use: Infusion, tincture, essential oil, incense

Lore: The ancient Romans named lavender after the word *lavare*, which means "to bathe." They were known to steep their bathwater with this plant, which was thought to be not only aromatic but also antiseptic.

Magickal Uses: Lavender can be used ritually for conjuring peaceful, soothing, and relaxing energies in your space. Create charms, try a ritual bath, or make a room spray to spritz over your linens and sheets to infuse your daily life with lavender's calming magick.

Easy Rituals, Potions, and Recipes: Create a tranquility-inducing herbal blend by combining dried lavender flowers and rose petals. Place a small amount in a burn-safe bowl. Use a lighter to light the blend of herbs and allow the sweet smoke to waft through the room, clearing any heavy energy from your space.

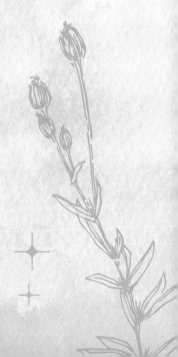

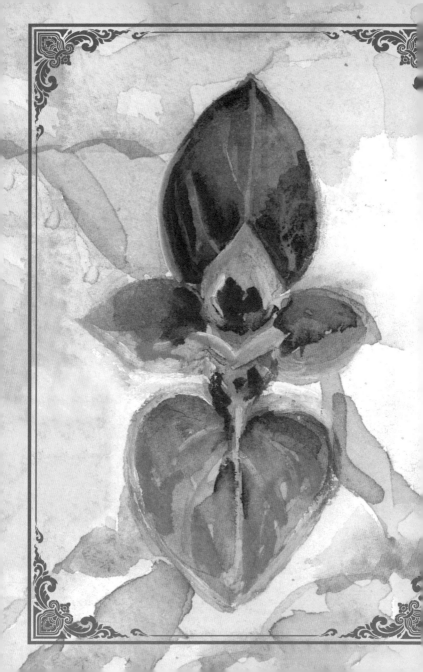

LEMON BALM

Melissa officinalis

Heart's Delight

Lemon balm, like its name suggests, has leaves that give off the scent of lemon. A member of the mint family, lemon balm is a bushy perennial growing up to 3 feet (1 m) tall, with heart-shaped leaves and small white flowers beloved by bees.

Parts Used: Leaves

Historical Medicinal Uses: Lemon balm has a long medicinal history and has been documented as a remedy for thousands of years. Greek physician Dioscorides recommended lemon balm leaves for bites and stings. It has also been used to treat colds, support the immune system, and aid digestion. With its delightful scent, lemon balm has been a popular herb to help balance mood and lift the spirits.

How to Use: Infusion, glycerite, tincture, tea

Lore: It's said that lemon balm is associated with Aphrodite and her priestesses, who were known as the Melissae. Beekeepers used lemon balm around hives to attract and calm bees. The fifteenth-century Swiss physician Paracelsus described lemon balm as the "elixir of life."

Magickal Uses: Because of its association with the goddess of love, lemon balm can be used in love drawing spells, rituals of self-love, and in ritual baths for soothing and support.

Easy Rituals, Potions, and Recipes: This magickal herb gets its name from the Greek word for "honeybee." To connect with bees in your green witch practice, cultivate lemon balm in your garden to attract these special and sacred pollinators. By caring for the lemon balm plant, you in turn care for and acknowledge the interconnected web of all things.

LEMONGRASS

Cymbopogon citratus

Fever Grass

Lemongrass is a tall, bushy herb in the grass family that is grown in tropical climates. The tall stalks and slender leaves have a lemony scent and are popular in cooking.

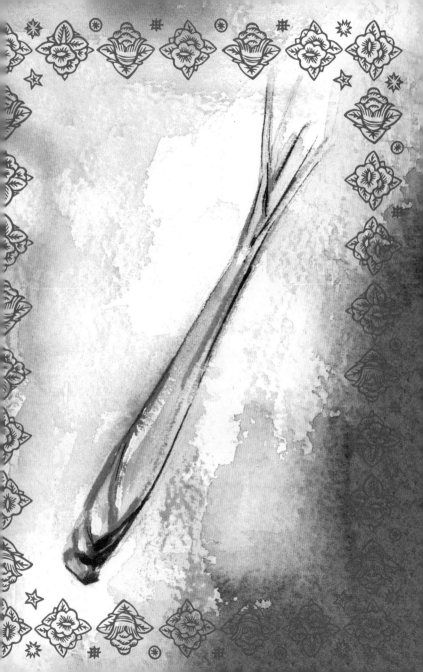

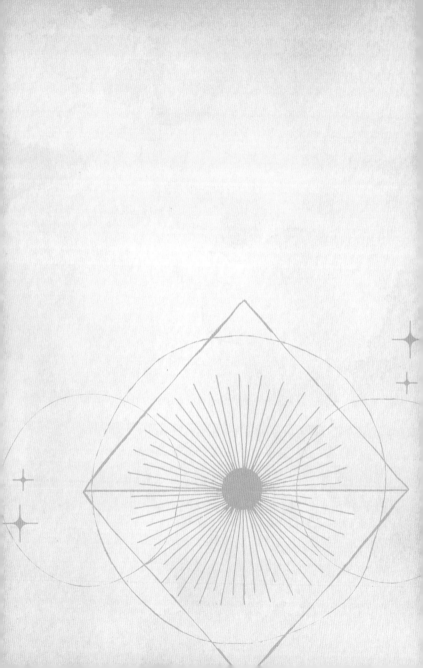

Parts Used: Whole plant

Historical Medicinal Uses: In East India and Sri Lanka, lemongrass has been historically used in a drink called fever tea. This brew was considered helpful not only for treating fevers but also as a tonic for overall well-being. Lemongrass oil is commonly used in aromatherapy.

How to Use: Essential oil, tea, incense

Lore: In India, folk wisdom holds that lemongrass's strong scent repels snakes; it may have a similar effect on other pests. In Celtic folklore, some legends tell that the Fae are drawn to lemongrass, and that cultivating it in your garden can support your relationship with the faerie world.

Magickal Uses: In magick, lemongrass is ideal for cleansing and purifying spells, and can also be used as an incense for smoke rituals.

Easy Rituals, Potions, and Recipes: Lemongrass makes for a wonderful DIY herbal bug spray. Fill a 4 ounce (115 ml) bottle with water, witch hazel, or vodka, then add about 50 to 75 total drops of lemongrass essential oil. Shake well. Before going outdoors, spray your bug repellent onto exposed skin or clothing (be sure to avoid your eyes and mucous membranes). Stored away from heat or sunlight, it will keep for six months.

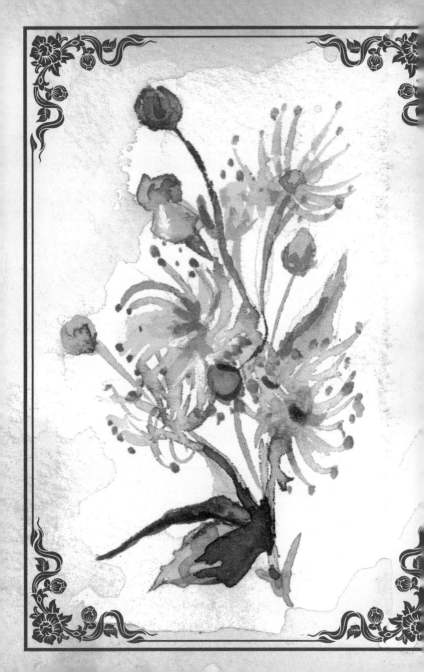

LINDEN

Tilia americana

Basswood

The American linden is a tall deciduous tree native to eastern North America. Lindens have gray-brown bark and pointy oval leaves. In summer, clusters of fragrant yellowish-white flowers droop down from their branches.

Parts Used: Leaves

Historical Medicinal Uses: In North America, some Indigenous peoples used linden to soothe digestive upsets. Historically it was also thought to be useful for anxiety relief, to calm feelings of restlessness and agitation.

How to Use: Infusion, tincture

Lore: The American linden is a relative of the European linden, which was associated with wisdom, compassion, and love as far back as the ancient Greeks. Thus the linden became a tree that is sacred to lovers. Marriage ceremonies were often performed under the shade of linden trees. Some lore suggests that lindens are also beloved by the Fae.

Magickal Uses: Linden works well in spells and rituals for love, divination, and release; linden is also useful in processing grief.

Easy Rituals, Potions, and Recipes: When you are dealing with a loss or are grieving, call on linden for support. An infusion of linden is ideal to sip for its supportive tenderness. You can also keep dried linden in a sachet, or simply tuck some under your pillow when you sleep.

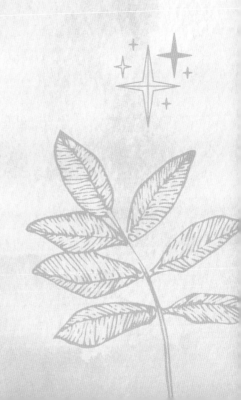

MARSHMALLOW

Althaea officinalis

The Cough Suppressant

Marshmallow can reach up to 7 feet (2.1 m) in height, with erect stems and short-stalked, cordate leaves that are velvety on both sides. The flowers are silky and pale pink in color, while the root is white.

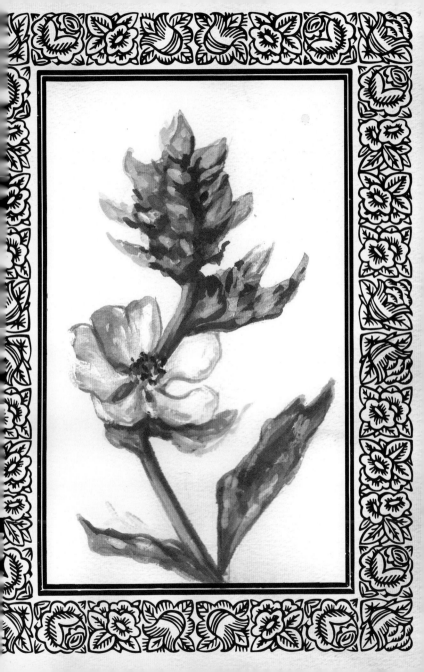

Parts Used: Roots

Historical Medicinal Uses: Its name comes from the Greek "to heal," and for good reason. Traditionally used as a poultice for inflammation, marshmallow can also be made into a tea for treating sore throats, GI issues, and urinary tract infections. The mucilage constituting this herb is widely known by herbalists as an effective remedy for cold, cough, and respiratory issues.

How to Use: Cold infusion, tincture, syrup, poultice; culinary uses

Lore: It has been said that during the Spanish Inquisition, potential victims of torture would paint their bodies with a concoction that included marshmallow sap, in an attempt to protect their skin from burns. In ancient Egypt, people enjoyed a marshmallow confection made from the roots of the mallow plant, which may be the first instance of marshmallow treats, though the herb is no longer used in the sweets we know as marshmallows today.

Magickal Uses: Marshmallow is commonly used as a protective and soothing herb in magick (much like its historical use in medicine!). Add it to candle dressings and spell bags for banishing and shielding against negative energy, or place on altars.

Easy Rituals, Potions, and Recipes: Decoct marshmallow root to use in herbal tea or add to your tea blend. Marshmallow root is also very popular for making homemade cough lozenges. The internet is full of different recipes, some dating back hundreds of years. Spend a crisp fall day embracing your kitchen witch and stocking up for the coming winter and the inevitable seasonal cough.

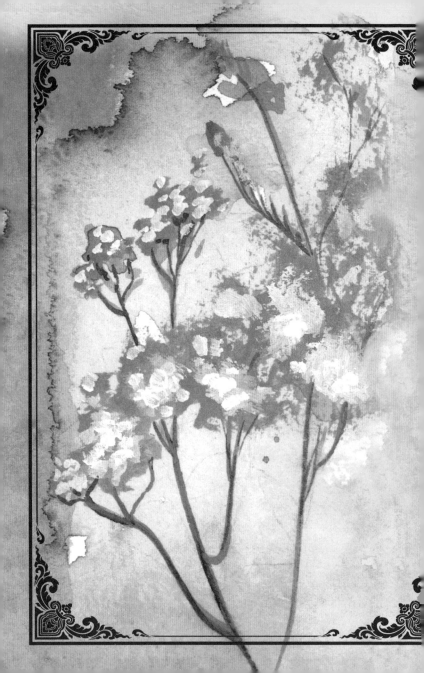

MEADOWSWEET

Filipendula ulmaria

Bridewort

A member of the rose family, meadowsweet is native to Europe and western Asia; however, it has been cultivated in North America. True to its name, it thrives in damp meadowlands. Growing 3-6 feet (1-2 m) tall, meadow-sweet stems are graced by clustered white flowers with a sweet scent.

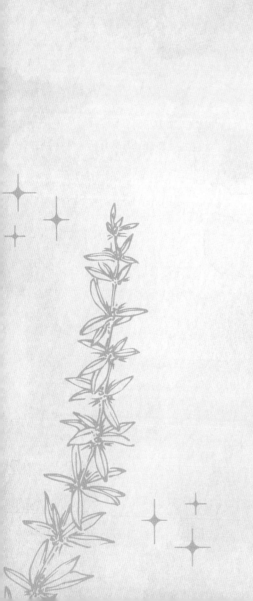

Parts Used: Aerial parts (all the parts above the soil)

Historical Medicinal Uses: Historically, meadowsweet was known as a natural painkiller and believed to reduce inflammation and swelling. Its pleasing aroma made it a popular strewing herb, and it was used in soothing baths.

How to Uses: Infusion, tincture, powder

Lore: Lore has it that meadowsweet was cultivated by the Druids for adding flavor to mead. Meadowsweet was said to have been a favorite of Queen Elizabeth I of England, who asked for it to be strewn on the floor of her chambers.

Magickal Uses: When performing ceremonies relating to love, marriage, or handfasting, call upon meadowsweet to foster eternal caring and commitment.

Easy Rituals, Potions, and Recipes: For wedding rituals, incorporate sprigs of meadowsweet into garlands and bouquets. It's also an excellent herb to include in love-drawing spells, charms, and baths.

MOTHERWORT

Leonurus cardiaca

Lion's Tail

Motherwort is a member of the mint family, originally from central Asia and southeastern Europe. It is now found globally and is also known as lion's ear or lion's tail. Motherwort is an upright perennial reaching approximately 3-5 feet (1-1.5 m) in height. Upright stems with green, sometimes purplish-tinged leaves are topped with small pink to purple flowers. The plant is often described as resembling a lion's tail.

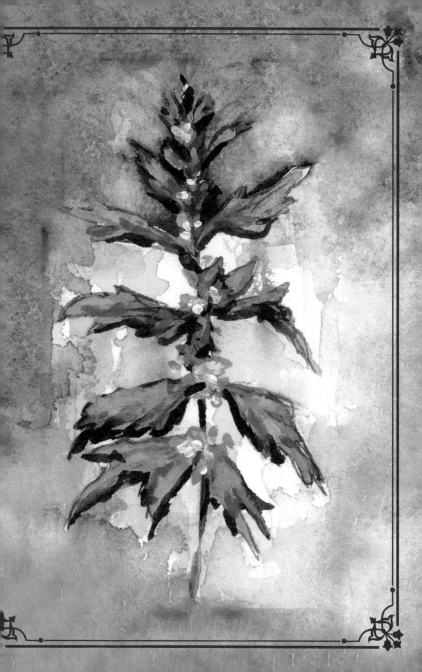

Parts Used: Leaves

Historical Medicinal Uses: Motherwort has long been used as a nervine, or support to the nervous system. It was also considered a wonderful ally to menstrual and uterine health, and was used in childbirth to reduce anxiety around the experience. The seventeenth-century English herbalist Nicholas Culpeper wrote that this herb "makes women joyful mothers of children and settles their wombs."

How to Use: Tincture, infusion

Lore: According to folklore, motherwort promotes longevity—legend tells of a town where motherwort grew plentifully on the banks of the river from which the town's water was drawn, and where the townspeople typically lived over a hundred years.

Magickal Uses: This lion-hearted herb can help support openness to the magick of the world. Call upon motherwort in ritual or magick when you need to feel strength, grace, and spiritual fortitude.

Easy Rituals, Potions, and Recipes: When you or your space feel haunted or hollow, make a charm of motherwort and keep it nearby, or hang a sprig in your home to give you courage and to hold your heart as it heals.

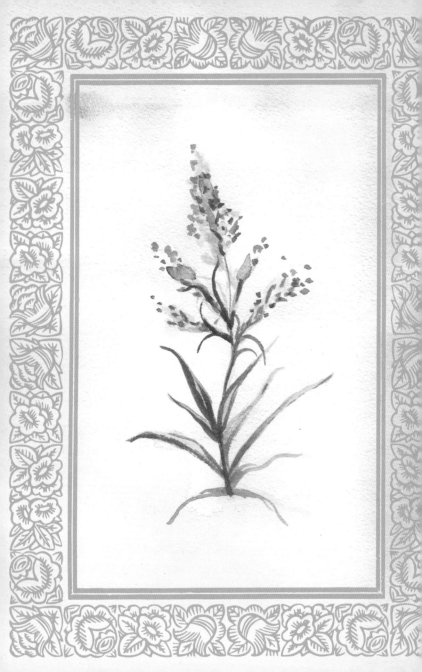

MUGWORT

Artemisia vulgaris

Ruled by Venus

Mugwort is considered by some people to be an invasive weed. This tall perennial thrives in uncultivated areas and can reach 3 feet (1 m) in height. It has a woody root, pinnate leaves with dense white hairs on their undersides and, often, a red-purple tint. Small florets produce dark-red or yellow petals. Mugwort is part of the ragweed family and like its cousins, can cause reactions in those with allergies.

Parts Used: Leaves, roots

Historical Medicinal Uses: Named after the ancient Greek goddess Artemis, the virginal huntress who presided over nature and childbirth, mugwort has been used to treat difficulties with menstruation, to promote smooth childbirth, and assist in expelling afterbirth. It is also a known nervine used to calm anxiety and ease depression. Mugwort is helpful as an overall tonic, and as a bitter, has played a part in many culinary traditions. It also has been burned as incense in different ceremonies.

How to Use: Tea, tincture, poultice, infusion, incense

Lore: During summer solstice or St. John's Eve ceremonies, a crown of mugwort was thought to protect against possession. In medieval Europe, the herb was used to flavor beer prior to hops.

Magickal Uses: Mugwort is considered a divinatory herb, and has long been used in lucid dreaming rituals or to enhance psychic ability. Taken as tea before bedtime, it is believed to awaken intuition and evoke vivid dreams. In ritual, it is burned as incense to aid in meditation or as a cleansing smudge.

Easy Rituals, Potions, and Recipes: Mugwort smoke is thought to assist in opening the third eye and promoting astral travel. To burn mugwort as incense, bundle a few dried stalks together to create a smoke stick, or place the loose leaves in an incense bowl with a charcoal disk. Another option is to add mugwort to an herb bundle. The smoke may also be helpful in opening the mind during meditation and when exploring past lives. Burning mugwort incense during spells and rituals can open and clear pathways of communication to your deities, spirits, and guides. In small amounts, dried mugwort can be added to a tea blend.

MULLEIN

Verbascum spp.

The Witch's Candle

Growing up to 8 feet (2.4 m) in height, mullein is recognizable by its hairy leaves that grow in a spiral shape. Tall spikes shoot up and produce small yellow flowers with five petals. In the first year of life, mullein produces a rosette of flowers, followed in the second year by a spike with a dense cluster of yellow flowers. Mullein is native to Asia, North Africa, and Europe, and has been cultivated widely.

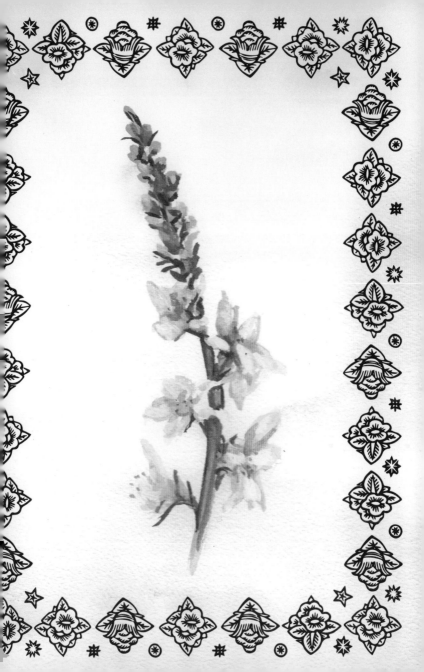

Parts Used: Leaves, flowers, root

Historical Medicinal Uses: Used in folk healing practices for centuries, this herb has been documented as a remedy for cramps, coughs, gout, and warts. It is commonly recognized by herbalists as an effective respiratory medicine, used to treat bronchitis, asthma, and other lung conditions; it may also be employed against ear infections.

How to Use: Tea, tincture, poultice, infusion, incense

Lore: In ancient Rome, mullein's large stalks made effective ceremonial torches. When dipped in tallow, mullein's trademark spike could carry a flame from place to place. During the California gold rush, mullein torches lined the mines to shed light as prospectors worked. As a magickal herb, it is believed to hold power over witches. Folklore says that mullein could help in retrieving children taken by the Fae.

Magickal Uses: Mullein is a protective herb. Add dried mullein leaves to dream pillows to ward off bad dreams, or hang sprigs in doorways for protection from negative energy.

Easy Rituals, Potions, and Recipes: Create your own ritual candles using mullein stalks as the wicks, or alternatively, burn the stalk itself as a candle. You can also use powdered mullein as a substitute in spells that call for earth or graveyard dirt.

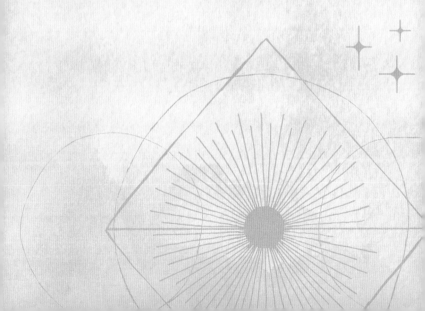

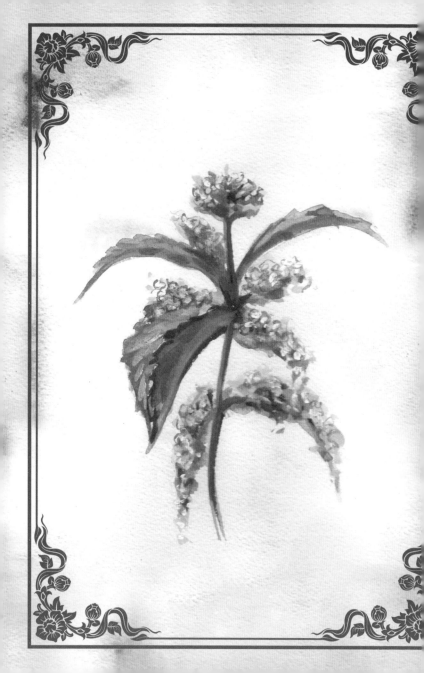

NETTLE

Urtica spp.

The Everyday Herb

Growing 2-6 feet (0.6-1.8 m) tall, nettle is notorious for the stinging hairs on its grooved stem and ovate dark-green leaves. It produces tiny green flowers. The stinging nettle is a favorite of herbalists. Originating in Europe, this plant now grows worldwide.

Parts Used: Stalks, leaves, rhizomes, seeds

Historical Medicinal Uses: Nettles are celebrated in traditional herbalism for their nutrient density and being rich in antioxidants as well as vitamins C and A. Featured in the writings of ancient Greek physician Hippocrates, nettle has long been recorded as a powerful nutritional tonic and as a nourishing food source. It has been used in many other ways, including to slow bleeding, treat seasonal allergies, soothe arthritic swelling, and even build milk supply in lactating mothers. This versatile and well-respected plant has earned its "everyday herb" nickname.

How to Use: Tea, tincture, juice, infusion; culinary uses

Lore: Burial shrouds made from nettle fibers have been found in Denmark dating five thousand years back. Stronger than cotton, nettle fibers have also been used to weave cordage for fishing nets. In folklore, thickets of nettle are said to indicate that the Fae are nearby. Interestingly, nettles can also be used as a protection against Fae magick.

Magickal Uses: It is no surprise that with their stinging leaves, nettles are used in work that enhances boundaries. Call on the energy of nettles in support of boundary magick.

Easy Rituals, Potions, and Recipes: Sprinkle dried nettle leaves in a circle around you when performing cord cutting and boundary spells. Call back your energy while the circle is open, then close it with the nettle, securing your energy safely inside.

OATSTRAW

Avena sativa

Common Oat

Oatstraw is a tall annual grass that originated in Asia, northwest Africa, and Europe, and today are grown worldwide in temperate regions. Oatstraw plants often reach 5 feet (1.5 m) in height with a single main stem and a cluster of green flowers. The grains or seeds are small, beige, and oval. The cereal most of us know as oats comes from the plant's ripened seeds, while the whole plant is oatstraw.

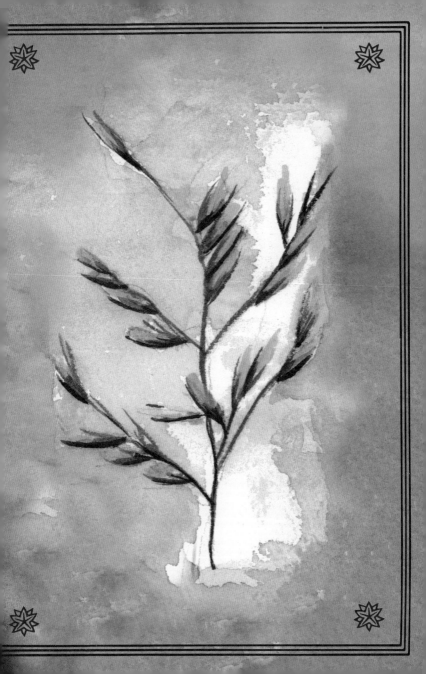

Parts Used: Whole plant

Historical Medicinal Uses: Among the oldest known and cultivated plants on earth, oat has a very long history as a medicinal herb. It is known as a soothing and supportive nervine historically used as a nourishing tonic to encourage overall relaxation and calm the nervous system. Hildegarde of Bingen, a nun and herbalist in the eleventh century, is said to have named oat as a "happiness herb." Oat was also commonly used to treat skin conditions and stomach problems.

How to Use: Infusion, tincture, glycerite

Lore: In ancient Greek mythology, legend has it that the deity Gaia, who represented the earth itself, was raised on milk from oats. Oat was also sacred to Demeter, goddess of the harvest.

Magickal Uses: Oatstraw is associated with wealth and abundance, making it ideal to work with in your rituals intended to draw in a bountiful harvest from whatever intention you set.

Easy Rituals, Potions, and Recipes: Make an abundance spell jar with oatstraw. You'll need an empty jar with a sealable top, a crystal that symbolizes abundance to you, and your intention, which you can write on a piece of paper and fold up. Put the crystal in the jar, and fill it with dried oatstraw to support your spell. Seal the jar and place it on an abundance altar or bury it in the earth somewhere safe.

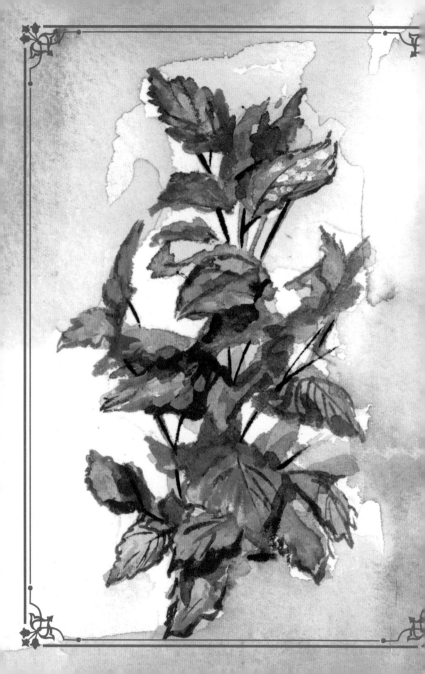

OREGANO

Origanum vulgare

Joy from the Mountain

Oregano is a member of the mint family, native to the Mediterranean, but now grown widely across the northern hemisphere. It is a flowering, shrubby perennial that grows 1-3 feet (0.3-1 m) tall, with dark-green aromatic leaves and small purple flowers.

Parts Used: Leaves

Historical Medicinal Uses: The ancient Greeks were big fans of this culinary herb, whose name roughly translated as "joy from the mountain." They would chew oregano leaves to ease the discomfort of toothaches. Oregano was also long touted as a remedy for indigestion, and in ancient Chinese medicine, as an anti-diarrheal.

How to Use: Tincture, glycerite, infusion, essential oil; culinary uses

Lore: Aphrodite, ancient Greek goddess of love, is said to have created oregano, which she grew in her garden on Mount Olympus. Long considered an antidote to poison, oregano also features in a legend about the Greek philosopher Aristotle, who is said to have noticed that tortoises who either ate or were bitten by snakes nibbled oregano leaves and suffered no ill effects.

Magickal Uses: Plant oregano near the door to your house or in window boxes to ward off negative energies. Tuck a sprig of oregano in your wallet to attract prosperity.

Easy Rituals, Potions, and Recipes: Because of its connection to the goddess Aphrodite, the ancient Greeks believed that drinking a love potion that included oregano, or even sleeping with a sprig of oregano under your pillow, would entice Aphrodite to whisper the name of your true love into your sleeping ear. For a modern take on this ancient spell, make a dream sachet with dried oregano leaves, a bit of lavender, and a few rose petals to thank the goddess for her support as you draw love in.

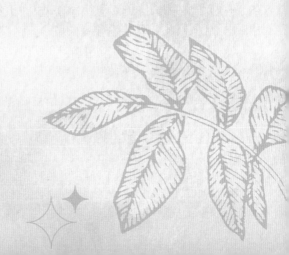

PASSIONFLOWER

Passiflora incarnata

Maypop

Passionflower is a climbing perennial vine with striking fringed white and purple flowers topped with orange berries commonly called maypops. Its unusual appearance makes the passionflower easy to spot, and gazing into its marvelous flowers is a magickal practice in and of itself. It originated in tropical climates but is cultivated widely.

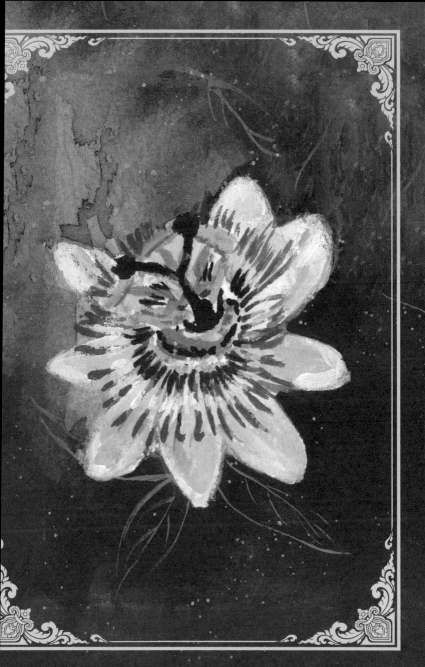

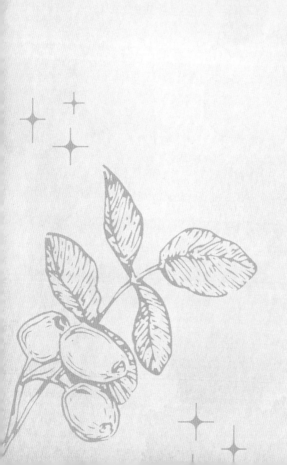

Parts Used: Leaves

Historical Uses: Historically, passionflower is known as a nervine herb, traditionally used for soothing tension and aiding in sleep. When restlessness is a symptom, passionflower is a strong herbal ally.

How to Use: Infusion, tea, tincture, glycerite

Lore: In fifteenth-century Spain, this plant became closely associated with the crucifixion of Jesus Christ. The spikes protruding from the center were said to symbolize the crown of thorns. In other cultures, passionflower represents a clock face.

Magickal Uses: In ritual and spellwork, passionflower is wonderful to work with when channeling or performing acts of divination. Call upon passionflower when you need support relaxing into your practice or the moment.

Easy Rituals, Potions, and Recipes: Make a tea from dried passionflower and sip before divining (it can be tarot, pendulums, spirit boards, or whatever practice calls to you). As you sip the tea, ask the passionflower to ease your anxieties and allow you to come into the present moment to be an open channel, ready to receive messages for your highest good.

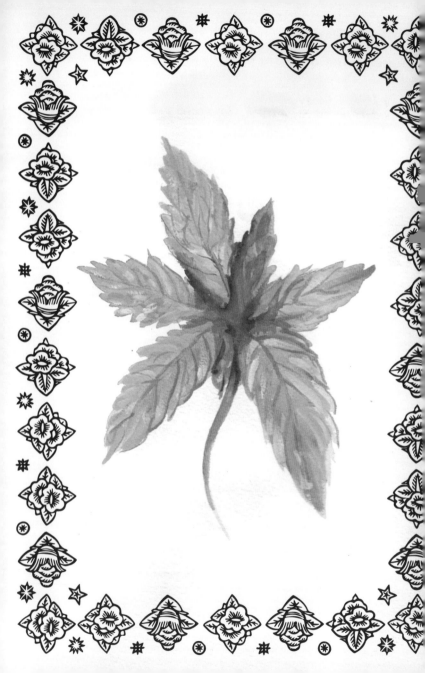

PEPPERMINT

Mentha piperita

The Ancient Herb

A cross between watermint and spearmint, peppermint grows up to 3 feet (1 m) in height. It has a square stem, and its pungent leaves are dark-green with reddish veins and a light fuzz. Purple flowers grow around the stem.

Parts Used: Leaves

Historical Medicinal Uses: Due to its volatile oil content, peppermint has traditionally been used as a digestive aid and remedy for bowel problems, flatulence, and indigestion. With its strong taste, peppermint is also a common flavoring herb in toothpaste, mouthwashes, and other edible products.

How to Use: Tea, tincture

Lore: Greek myths tell how Hades, god of the underworld, seduced the nymph Minthe, causing his wife, Persephone, to became enraged with jealousy and turn Minthe into a plant that people would constantly walk on. Outraged, Hades imbued the plant with a wonderful scent, ensuring those who stepped on it would smell the enticing aroma and remember Minthe and her beauty.

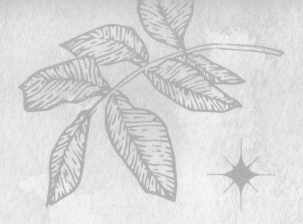

Magickal Uses: Dress a red candle in peppermint oil for use in love spells and sex magick.

Easy Rituals, Potions, and Recipes: Blend some peppermint, lavender, passion flower, and skullcap together for a relaxing evening tea. Drink after dinner for extra digestive support. Create a stimulating peppermint body oil by infusing the herb into a carrier oil, such as sweet almond, for use in massage and sensual touch.

Pipsissewa

Chimaphila umbellata

The King's Cure

This evergreen shrub found throughout the northern hemisphere produces shiny, bright leaves arranged in opposite pairs of three or four along the stem, with fair hairs along the tooth ends. Flowers are pink or white and grow in umbels, followed by a fruit in the late summer.

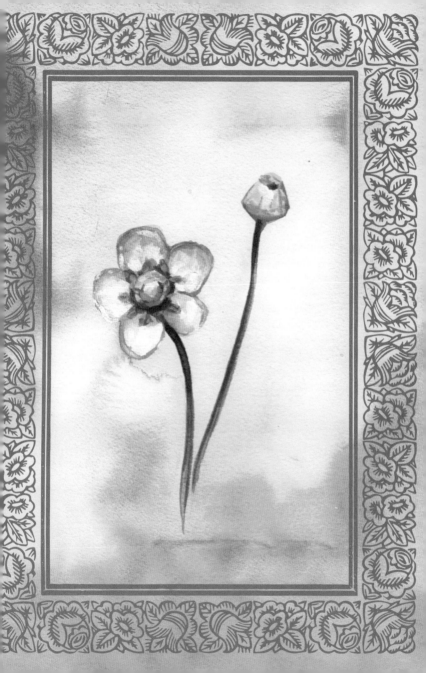

Parts Used: Leaves

Historical Medicinal Uses: Historically, pipsissewa was used by Indigenous peoples or the Americas as a diuretic and a tonic for kidney and bladder issues. Also known as a fever reducer, it worked by inducing sweating. Additionally, pipsissewa was thought to be helpful with respiratory complaints. Some native peoples used pipsissewa to treat skin conditions such as rashes or bug bites. In Europe, it was used to treat tuberculosis, also known as "the king's evil," giving the herb its nickname of "the king's cure."

How to Use: Tea, tincture, poultice

Lore: Pipsissewa's main claim to fame was as a flavoring in old-time root beer recipes. It was also used in homemade candies.

Magickal Uses: In magickal ritual, pipsissewa is believed to be useful in calling spirits and promoting prosperity.

Easy Rituals, Potions, and Recipes: Add dried pipsissewa leaves to a sachet with a piece of raw citrine to draw in abundance and material wealth.

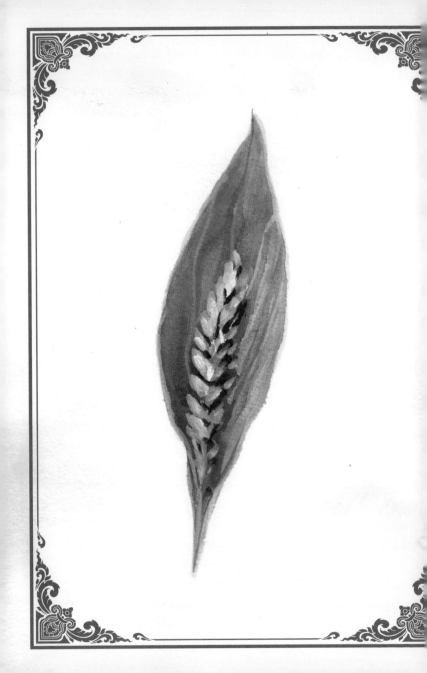

PLANTAIN

Plantago lanceolata or P. major

The Soldier's Herb

Also known as broadleaf plantain (not to be confused with the banana-like fruit), plantain has a basal rosette of oval leaves that are hairless and have a smooth margin. A central spike shoots up with tiny greenish-brown flowers that have a purple stamen and cluster around the shooting spike. Small brown fruits appear in late summer and fall; plantain seeds are tiny and blown by the wind. It grows widely in Europe, Asia, and North America, where it is found along roadsides and fields, often considered a weed.

Parts Used: Leaves, roots, seeds

Historical Medicinal Uses: A popular herb among healers as far back as ancient Greeks and Persians, plantain was historically used as an effective remedy for many skin issues, including cuts, scrapes, burns, bites, stings, and sunburns. It was also commonly used by herbalists as a diuretic, and to treat respiratory concerns.

How to Use: Tea, tincture, poultice, salve, infusion, wash, syrup

Lore: Plantain has been referred to as "nature's Band-Aid" for its versatile uses. It was used as a wound dressing on the battlefield, earning it the name "soldier's herb." Among Indigenous North American peoples, it was known as the "white man's footprint," since its seeds were literally carried on the heels of shoes and the plants sprouted up where European colonizers had settled.

Magickal Uses: Plantain is an herb associated with personal growth, confidence, and courage. It is excellent for use in protection spells and in times when you need to call back your energy.

Easy Rituals, Potions, and Recipes: Fashion a bundle of plantain leaves into a bouquet and hang it above your doorways or on your altar for protection. For confidence, pack a small bundle or pieces of leaves into a jar or tin and take with you when needed.

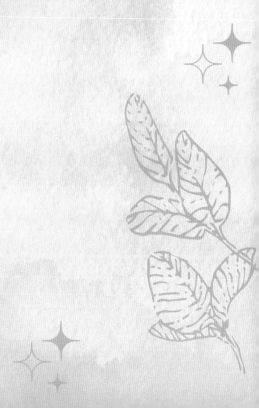

RED CLOVER

Trifolium pratense

Meadow Trefoil

Red clover is a flowering plant in the bean family. With leaves that have a distinctive triplet shape, red clover is beloved by bumblebees, which are often seen visiting the clover's bristlelike pink flower. It is native to Europe, western Asia, and northwest Africa, but has naturalized widely around the world.

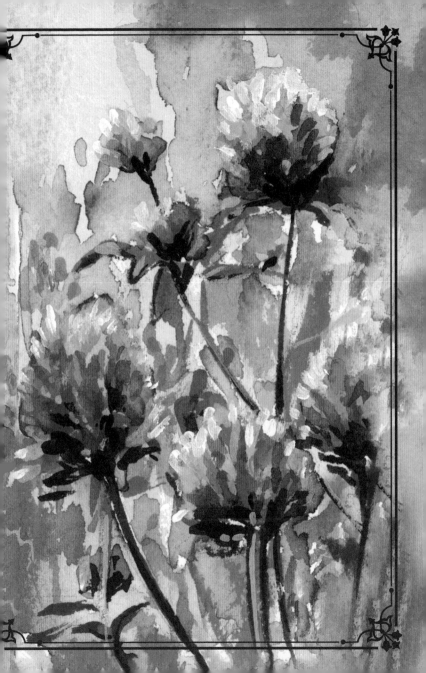

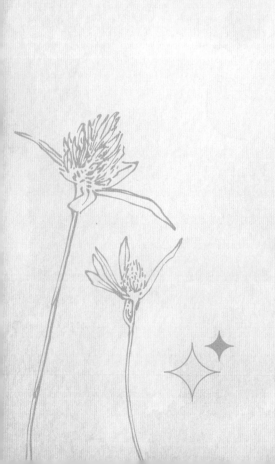

Parts Used: Flowers

Historical Medicinal Uses: A staple in many healing traditions, including Ayurvedic and traditional Chinese medicine, red clover has been used to move lymph, as an immune system tonic, and to support endocrine function.

How to Use: Infusion, tincture, glycerite, incense

Lore: According to Greek and Roman mythology, the three-leaved plant was associated with the triple goddesses—Artemis, Selene, and Hecate—who were connected to the female, the moon, and magick.

Magickal Uses: Red clover is an ideal herb to use during rituals intended to connect to your goddess or when initiating an open call for goddess connection.

Easy Rituals, Potions, and Recipes: Create a goddess invocation incense of red clover tops by blending with rosemary, mugwort, and bay leaf. Crush the dried herbs together and burn over a charcoal disk at the beginning of any goddess work. Burn the blend on your altar daily to call in your deity.

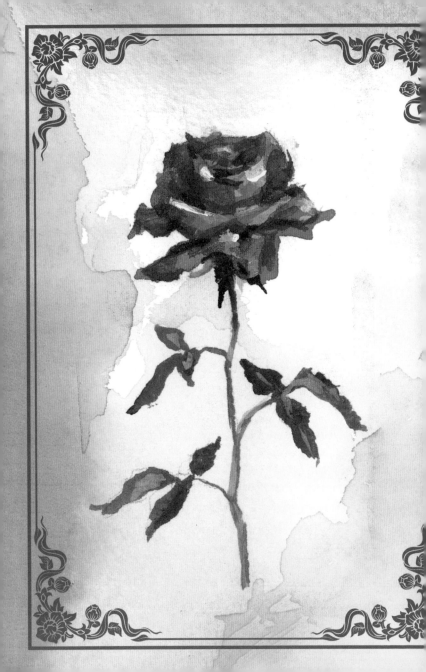

ROSE

Rosa sp.

Queen of the Flowers

An ancient flowering shrub noted for its exceptional flowers often protected by thorny stems, the rose has more than three hundred species (and thousands of cultivars) and grows throughout the northern hemisphere. It may have originally been cultivated in ancient China. As varied as it is beautiful, the rose takes climbing, trailing, and upright forms, and flowers come in a range of colors, some scented.

Parts Used: Petals

Historical Medicinal Uses: Historically, rose has had many uses in traditional herbal and folk medicines around the world, from soothing the stomach to tending to a frayed nervous system. Ancient writings attest to the power of a rose-petal sitz bath to support the female reproductive system, the use of rose-infused rinses for mouth sores, and of course the powerful scent of rose as a perfume.

How to Use: Infusion, tincture, capsule, tea, essential oil

Lore: Rose has been honored for thousands of years. It is associated with the Greek goddess Aphrodite, who, it was said, created the red rose from a drop of her own blood. Rose was also a favorite of Egyptian queen Cleopatra, who is said to have strewn rose petals about her palace so that her lover Marc Antony would always think of her upon smelling a rose.

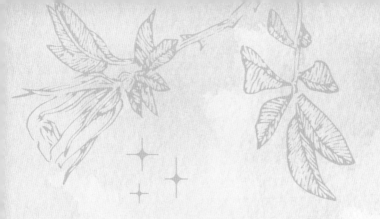

Magickal Uses: It's no surprise that rose petals are used in spells and rituals for attraction, romance, and self-love. Working with rose's connection to love and sensuality, call on these soft petals for ritual baths, oils, anointing candles, or creating spell jars and sachets.

Easy Rituals, Potions, and Recipes: Glamour magick uses items like perfumes, jewelry, oils, makeup, or clothing to cast a spell. It can support you in a spell of protection or in attracting abundance, manifesting intentions, or influencing and transmuting energy. It can also help you connect with your own body and aura; it is a magickal way to practice presence and celebrate preparing and setting intentions for the day. Make a rose-petal blush and call upon glamour magick as you apply it daily. Rinse roses thoroughly in water, dry them upside down for two weeks, then grind the roses into a fine powder to create a natural blush (some folks add cornstarch as well). As you pat it onto your cheekbones, cast a spell of attraction and self-love.

ROSEMARY

Salvia rosmarinus

Herb of Remembrance

Rosemary is an evergreen shrub that can grow 3-6 feet (1-2 m) high. Its leaves are gray-green and needlelike in shape and have a strong aroma. Flowers are tiny and may be white, purple, blue, or pink. Rosemary is native to the Mediterranean region but is widely cultivated as a popular culinary herb.

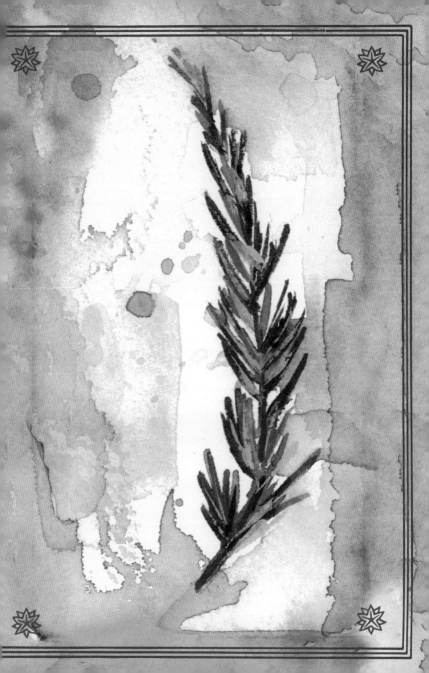

Parts Used: Leaves, twigs, oil

Historical Medicinal Uses: Rosemary has a long history of medicinal use in cultures ranging from ancient China to medieval Europe, and has been used to treat colds, sore throats, and fever. It was also considered a digestive-supporting herb (and of course was a favorite in culinary magick!).

How to Use: Infusion, tincture, glycerite, capsule, topical, incense; culinary uses

Lore: Rosemary is associated with remembrance. In ancient Greece, scholars would wear a garland of rosemary around their heads to improve their memory while studying. Medieval healers burned rosemary to ward off contagion.

Magickal Uses: Rosemary is a good choice for use in spellwork and charms to support general health, for clearing negative energy, and in protection rituals. A symbol of love and loyalty, it is often incorporated into handfasting ceremonies. Rosemary can also be called upon in fertility magick.

Easy Rituals, Potions, and Recipes: When practicing ancestor veneration, honor, or worship, burn a bit of dried rosemary in a fire-safe container and allow the rosemary's sweet smoke to envelop your altar. A way of enhancing remembrance, burning rosemary can help you to connect with those who are no longer in their physical bodies.

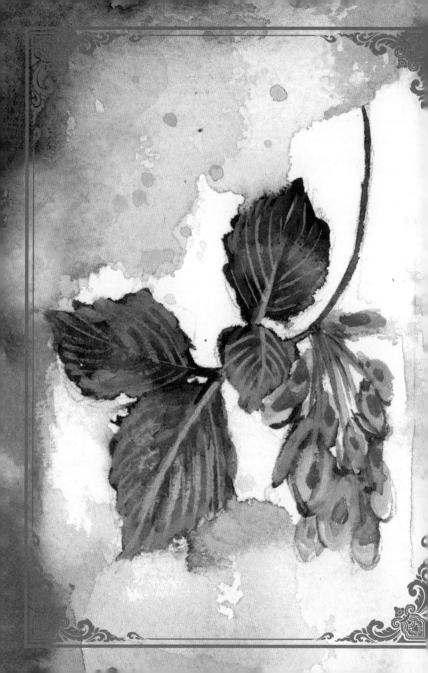

SLIPPERY ELM

Ulmus rubra

Moose Elm

The slippery elm is native to eastern North America. One of the smaller members of the elm family, it grows 50-60 feet (15-18 m) in height. It has a flat-topped crown and long branches; some describe its outer bark as coarse-textured, while its inner bark has a mucus that led to its common name. Slippery elm leaves are broad with teeth around the edges.

Parts Used: Bark

Historical Medicinal Uses: The Indigenous peoples of North America used slippery elm in traditional medicine in a number of ways, including to add moisture to tissues, to support irritated tissues (especially in the digestive tract), as a healing salve, and as a cough and cold support. Slippery elm is endangered due to overharvesting and Dutch elm disease, so use sparingly and be sure to regenerate.

How to Use: Infusion, capsules, topical

Lore: Elms have a long association with magick. In ancient Greek tales, the hero Orpheus rescued his wife Eurydice from the underworld, and where he played his harp, an elm tree grew. Anglo-Saxon folklore held that elm trees were the favorite of wood elves.

Magickal Uses: In alignment with its medicinal properties, think of slippery elm when you're looking to add
ease or flow to your spells. Many find slippery elm of assistance in communication spells, whether to bolster a pub-
lic speaking engagement or to block gossip, allowing the
unkind words to slide right off.

Easy Rituals, Potions, and Recipes: Because slippery
elm is an at-risk tree, instead of incorporating it in a recipe
or spell in its physical form, try to connect with its energy.
One way to do this is by meditating near or under a slippery elm (if you don't have one nearby, you can picture it
in your mind), and see what messages it may have for you!

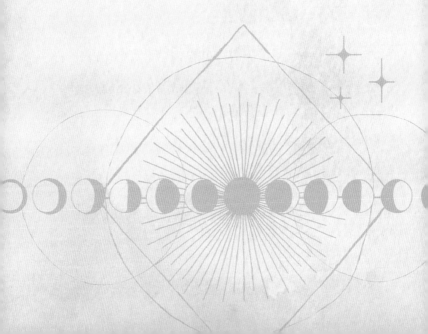

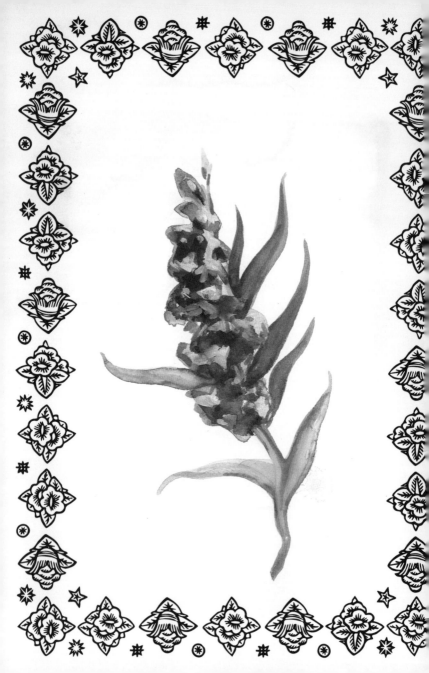

SKULLCAP

Scutellaria spp.

The Relaxing Herb

Skullcap is a flowering perennial in the mint family, native to northern Europe, Canada, and Asia. It is a branching plant that grows up to 3 feet (1 m) tall, with green leaves arranged in opposite pairs along the square stem. Skullcap flowers have a helmetlike shape, and their scientific name translates from the Latin word *scutella*, which means "little dish." The small, hooded flowers are purplish-blue in color.

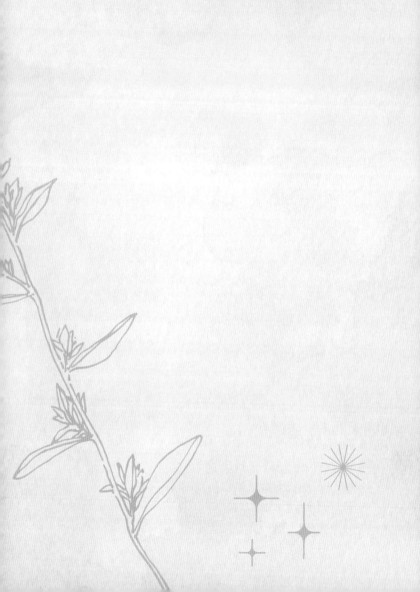

Parts Used: Leaves, flowers, stems

Historical Medicinal Uses: Skullcap was historically used by Indigenous North American peoples to stimulate menstruation, relieve breast pain, and help expel afterbirth. It has long been regarded as a powerful nervine and an important calming plant for herbalists treating nervous disorders and insomnia. Skullcap has also been used throughout history to treat stomach ailments and chronic pain.

How to Use: Tea, tincture

Lore: A doctor in 1772 claimed to have cured four hundred people and one thousand cattle of rabies using skullcap, giving it the nickname of "mad dog," but his claims were later debunked.

Magickal Uses: In alignment with its traditional medicinal profile as a nervine herb, skullcap can be used as a soothing ally in magick and ritual. If your spell calls for a bit of calming or de-escalation, call on skullcap.

Easy Rituals, Potions, and Recipes: Blend a calming before-bedtime tea using skullcap, passionflower, lavender, and rose.

St. John's Wort

Hypericum perforatum

The Happy Herb

St. John's wort is a bushy perennial that grows 1-3 feet (0.3-1 m), with branching stems and pale-green oblong leaves. It produces cheerful, bright-yellow, five-petaled flowers covered in tiny black dots that release red oil. St. John's wort is native to Europe, north Africa, and western Asia, but is now found all over the world.

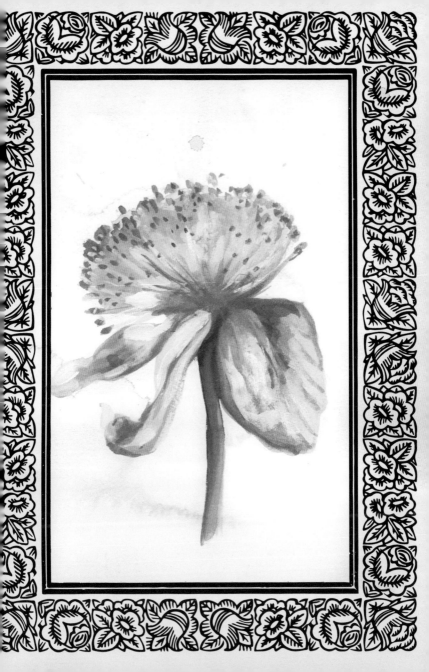

Parts Used: Leaves, flowers

Historical Medicinal Uses: With documented use dating back thousands of years to the ancient Greek healers, St. John's wort has long been commonly used to lift the spirits, fight depression, and treat anxiety. It is also a known plant medicine for treating skin irritations and promoting wound healing. St. John's wort has also been used to alleviate menstrual cramping and symptoms of menopause.

How to Use: Tea, tincture, poultice, salve, infusion

Lore: Named after St. John the Baptist, it is said the red sap "bleeds" in August on the day the saint was beheaded. Legend has it that St. John's wort received its name because it bloomed at the time of the Feast of St. John the Baptist in June, near the summer solstice.

Magickal Uses: Work with St. John's wort when you want to connect with your inner sunshine. It can bring a feeling of brightness to any ritual. Call on its positive energies when you are in need of its rays of light.

Easy Rituals, Potions, and Recipes: Create a tincture of St. John's wort to take whenever you need a little liquid sunshine. Simply fill a mason jar ⅔ full of the dried herb and cover with vodka until the jar is full. (Leave a little room for shaking!) Screw on the lid and place the jar in a dark cabinet for one full moon cycle, or thirty days, shaking every day or two. When the cycle is complete, strain the liquid into a glass jar with a dropper for future use. Return the spent herbs to the earth, thanking them for their healing magick.

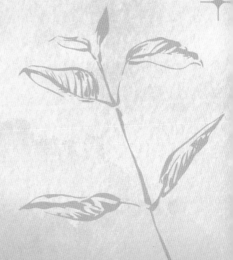

TURMERIC

Curcuma longa

The Golden Spice

Turmeric is a member of the ginger family. A perennial with grasslike leaves and greenish-yellow flowers, turmeric is native to southeast Asia. Strictly speaking, turmeric is the underground part of the plant known as the rhizome. When turned into a powder, turmeric is a beautiful orange color.

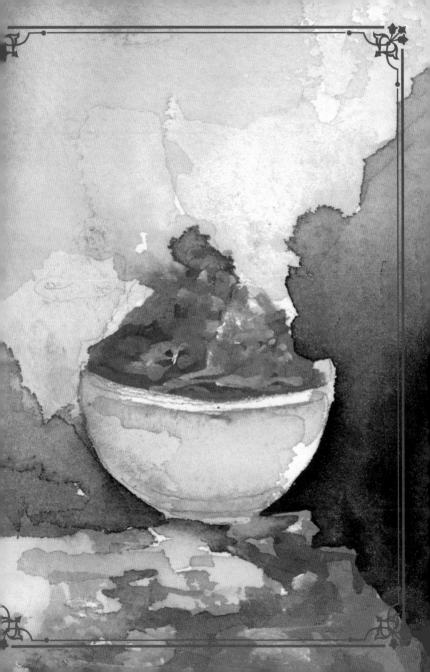

Parts Used: Rhizome

Historical Medicinal Uses: Used in multiple cultures for thousands of years in medicine, for culinary practices, and as a dye, turmeric was a staple of Ayurvedic healing, used to support those struggling with complaints from arthritis to digestive issues, and also as an invigorating and warming spice.

How to Use: Decoction, tincture, capsule, powder, dye

Lore: Said to have been grown in the legendary Hanging Gardens of Babylon, turmeric features in many ancient practices. According to folk tradition in southern India, the rhizome, when worn as a charm, can ward off evil and call in protective and supportive energies. An old Hindu wedding tradition is to wear a yellow necklace dyed with turmeric paste.

Magickal Uses: Call upon the vibrant energy of turmeric for spells of healing and vitality.

Easy Rituals, Potions, and Recipes: Make a ritual plant dye using turmeric, ideally on a natural fabric such as raw silk. Dye an altar cloth, ribbons, or other materials that you might use in ritual to infuse your magick with a bit of turmeric's energy. Another great way to use turmeric is to work with its vibrant orange in color magick.

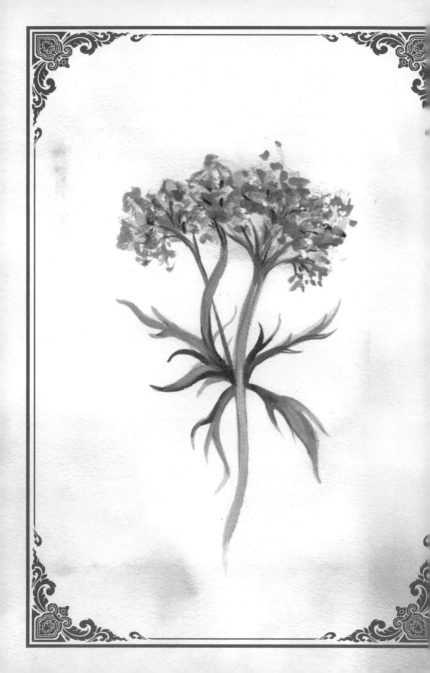

Valerian

Valeriana officinalis

The Liminal Herb

Valerian is a perennial that can grow to 3 feet (1 m) tall, with divided pinnate leaves and small white to pale-pink flowers. Although native to Europe and Asia, it is now grown widely around the world.

Parts Used: Rhizome, roots

Historical Medicinal Uses: With its use dating back to ancient Greece, valerian (from the Latin word *valere* or "strength" is a popular healing herb. Traditionally used as a calming sleep aid due to its light sedative properties, valerian is also recognized as a useful plant for treating anxiety and calming the nerves. (Note that for a small number of people, valerian is known to have an energizing effect instead of its usual calming qualities.)

How to Use: Tea, tincture, incense

Lore: A popular herb in Samhain and Yule celebration rituals, valerian is believed to ward off evil and, probably due to its ability to induce sleepiness, aid in traveling to the liminal spaces. In medieval Sweden, it was sometimes used in wedding celebrations, tucked into the clothing of the groom to ward off the envy of elves. Folklore says that if you put valerian under your tongue before kissing the person of your dreams, they will fall in love with you in return. During World War II, it was sometimes given to ease the effects of shell shock (now known as PTSD).

Magickal Uses: In magick, valerian is known as a peaceful plant. When your ritual or spell is focused on soothing distress, creating harmony, or bringing tranquility to a situation, call on valerian.

Easy Rituals, Potions, and Recipes: Use dried valerian root as an incense by sprinkling it on a smoldering charcoal disk to increase awareness and assist in travel to the astral and liminal planes. Blend with mugwort for an especially potent opener to the other realms.

Vitex

Vitex agnus-castus

Chaste Tree Berry

As a shrub, vitex may grow to 3 feet (1 m), but as a tree, this fast-grower can reach 22 feet (almost 7 m) in height, with palm-shaped, dark-green leaves that are silvery on the underside. Its foliage is aromatic. In summer, it produces small purple flowers that grow in panicles, and small gray berries.

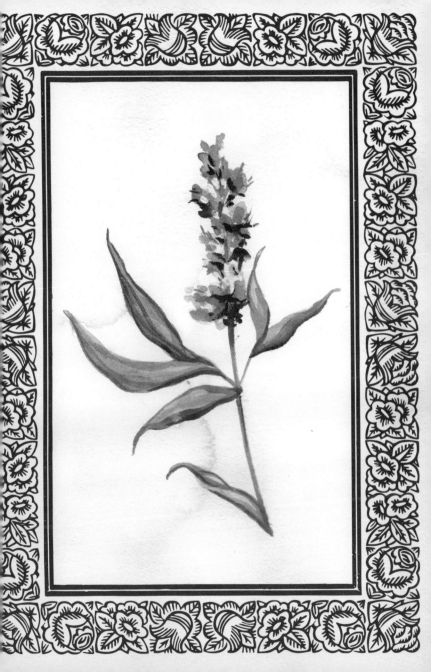

Parts Used: Berry

Historical Medicinal Uses: A plant medicine known for treating women's issues, vitex has a long history of use for menstrual cramps, hormonal changes, dysmenorrhea, and promoting fertility.

How to Use: Tea, tincture, incense

Lore: Long associated with chastity, the vitex earned the common name "chaste berry" because ingesting it reportedly reduced sexual desire. In ancient Rome, the Vestal Virgins carried vitex branches to symbolize sexual purity. It was also taken by monks in the Middle Ages to promote chastity.

Magickal Uses: With its deep connection to the womb and women's history, vitex can be called upon in rituals connected to the divine feminine or those intended for healing ancestral trauma.

Easy Rituals, Potions, and Recipes: Create a botanical cleansing stick by drying and bundling the stalks and flowers of vitex. Light the end with a match and cleanse yourself and your space with the smoke.

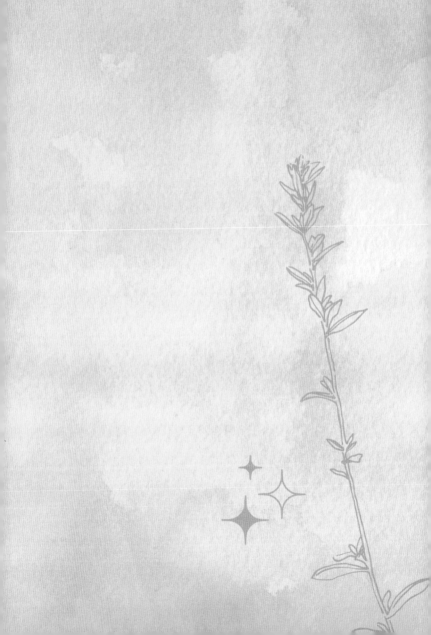

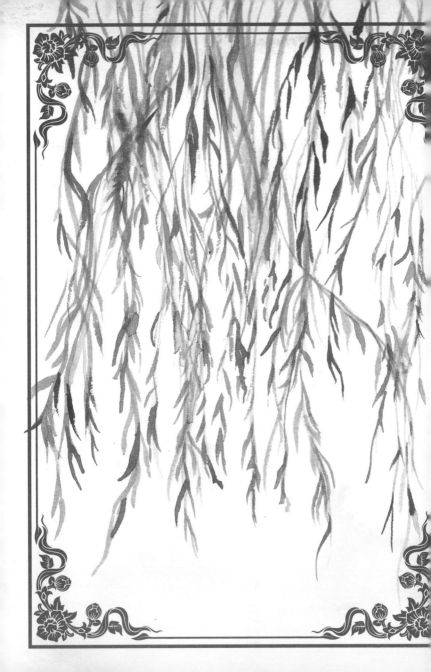

WHITE WILLOW

Salix alba

The Witch's Wand

White willow is a large deciduous tree that grows 10-32 yards (9-29 m) tall, with rough gray-brown bark. Green leaves have fine, silky white hairs on the underside, giving them a whitish cast, leading to the common name. Willow is often found growing near water.

Parts Used: Bark, leaves, roots

Historical Medicinal Uses: Possibly the oldest analgesic in herbal medicine, willow bark has been used to treat pain in various areas of the body for many centuries, with records dating back to ancient Chinese, Greek, and Egyptian healers. Preparations made from willow bark were used to ease discomfort from headaches, cramps, and arthritis, and it was chewed to relieve tooth and mouth pain. Willow was additionally used to lower fevers, and led to the development of the original aspirin.

How to Use: Tea, tincture

Lore: Sacred to several of the ancient Greek goddesses, including Hecate and Persephone, willow was associated with water. Orpheus brought willow on his journey to the underworld, and the tree has since been associated with poetry. In Celtic folklore, the willow was associated with grief. In medieval times, those who had been scorned or rejected by a lover may have worn a crown or garland made of willow to ease their bitterness. The willow's branches were said to make powerful wands for witches.

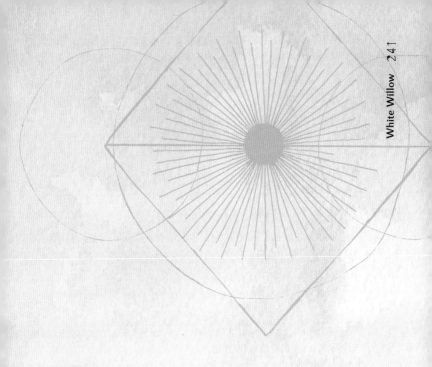

Magickal Uses: Willow is known to be a powerful healer of damaged or weary spirits and can be used in spells that call for fortification of emotion and inner strength.

Easy Rituals, Potions, and Recipes: Create your own wand for use in ritual by collecting the thin, fallen branches of a willow tree. Bundle them together with twine to create a sturdy wand. Affix a clear quartz point to the end to direct the energy. Decorate with colorful ribbons, flowers, or any other tokens of your craft that speak to you.

Witch Hazel

Hamamelis virginiana

Winter's Bloom

A deciduous tree or shrub that often tops out around 10 feet (3 m) in height, the witch hazel is native to eastern North America. It is often found in mountainous woodlands, where it is easily spotted with its clusters of yellow flowers that bloom during fall and winter.

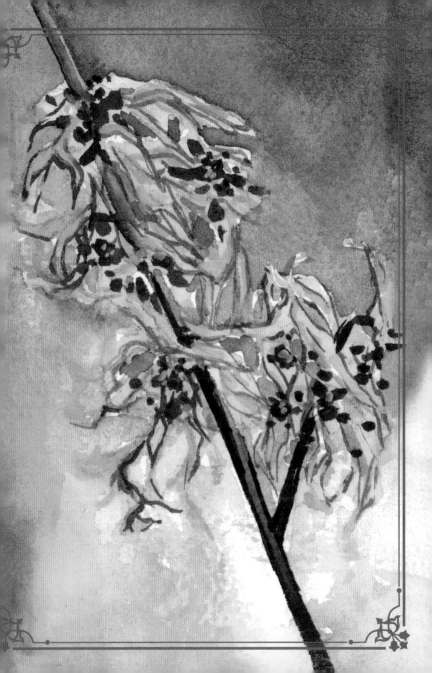

Parts Used: Bark, leaves

Historical Medicinal Uses: With its astringent properties, witch hazel is historically famous for tending to topical irritations. Herbalists have long used it for eye troubles and inflammation, acne, insect bites, and even sensitive scalps.

How to Use: Topical uses, tincture

Lore: Folklore says that the Mohegan peoples, indigenous to the US east coast, showed the English how to use witch hazel sticks to dowse for water. It is said that witch hazel gets its name from the Middle English *wicke* meaning "lively," and *wych* from the Anglo-Saxon for "bend" (referring to the practice of dowsing itself).

Magickal Uses: Call on witch hazel to banish negative energies or when you want to eliminate something that no longer serves you from your life, whether it is a relationship that is not working or a goal that you have outgrown.

Easy Rituals, Potions, and Recipes: Enjoy a cleansing ritual bath to banish negativity, bad memories, or other unwanted emotions. Fill your bath with warm water and add witch hazel (you can also add Epsom salts). After your soak, as the water drains away, focus on the departure of the feelings you no longer want, letting them swirl away with the water.

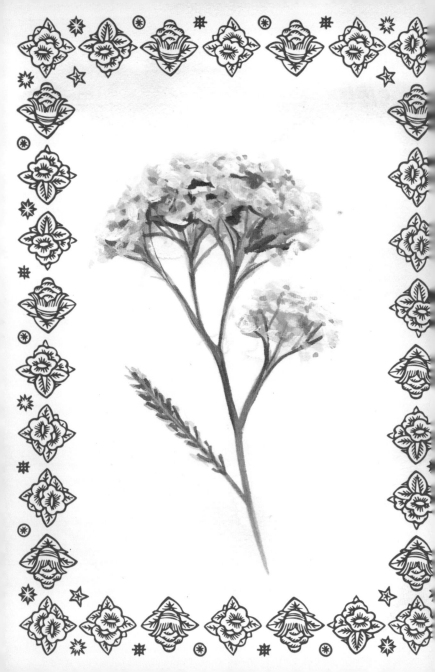

YARROW

Achillea millefolium

Soldier's Woundwort

An erect perennial in the aster family, yarrow has multiple, even-leaved stems topped with flat, tightly packed clusters of flower heads that may be white, yellow, or pink. Yarrow is sometimes called plumajillo, meaning "little feather," due to the shape of its leaves. Other common names are devil's nettle, sanguinary, milfoil, and thousand seal.

Parts Used: Aerial parts (all the parts above the soil)

Historical Medicinal Uses: Widely recognized for its wound-healing properties, yarrow's Latin name comes from the ancient Greek warrior Achilles, who was taught by the centaur Chiron to use it for treating battle wounds. Throughout history, yarrow was commonly used on battlefields as an effective treatment to slow bleeding, promote healing, and prevent infection. Yarrow is also considered by herbalists to be a useful plant for treating cold and respiratory issues, and it has digestive use as a bitter.

How to Use: Tea, tincture, poultice

Lore: In the Middle Ages, yarrow was believed to aid both in summoning the devil and driving him away, making it a popular herb for use in Christian exorcisms. Yarrow dries well and has long been used in bouquets.

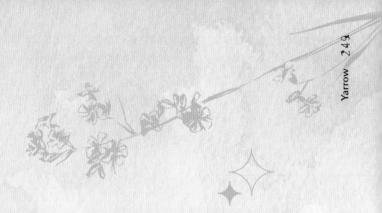

Magickal Uses: In magick, yarrow has often been used as a protective herb. Carry yarrow, or hang it in your doorway to call on its protective properties. It is also used in love and protection spells.

Easy Rituals, Potions, and Recipes: To send a magickal message to a loved one, simply write the words on a piece of paper with intent. When finished, sprinkle yarrow on the paper and fold three times. Burn the paper and the herbs inside in a red or pink candle, focusing as the smoke sends your message to the universe and your intended recipient.

YELLOW DOCK

Rumex crispus

Curly Dock

A member of the buckwheat family, yellow dock is a small, leafy plant with yellow-brown roots and a branched stem that grows up to 3 feet (1 m) in height, with clusters of flowers. Its lance-shaped leaves are slightly ruffled, giving it the nickname "curly dock." This flowering plant is native to Europe and western Asia, but grows widely in a variety of habitats. In some places it is considered invasive.

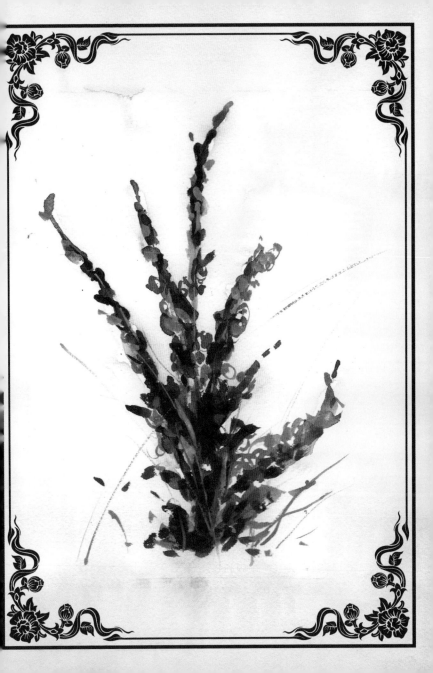

Parts Used: Leaves, root

Historical Medicinal Uses: Yellow dock has been traditionally used as a remedy for skin conditions, as well as a diuretic, tonic, liver support, and gentle laxative. Herbalists recognize this herb as a potent plant medicine for iron deficiencies. In historical herbalism, yellow dock has also been called upon to ease pain and swelling and as an overall wellness tonic. Some believe it can also treat a variety of infections.

How to Use: Tea, tincture, poultice, salve, wash

Lore: In Gaelic lore, it is thought that if the faeries possessed a child, yellow dock could break their hold and release the afflicted child. Some European cultures believed yellow dock could bring prosperity, and shopkeepers were known to boil the roots and then rub the water on the doors of their businesses to draw in customers.

Magickal Uses: Yellow dock promotes movement in the body, so it may be used magickally to support flow; call on yellow dock to break through emotional blockages and clear the way.

Easy Rituals, Potions, and Recipes: To create a yellow dock wash, boil the herb for five minutes and let simmer for fifteen more. Strain the water into a jar for future use. Thank the spent herb for its assistance in your craft, and return it to the earth. Use the wash on surfaces as needed to attract abundance and create clear pathways.

ABOUT THE AUTHORS

Shelby Bundy is the creator and owner of Tamed Wild, which she created in 2016 as a brand of herbal medicines and concoctions designed to support those in search of alternatives to modern medicine. Today, Tamed Wild sells a range of natural apothecary products—from herbs to teas, and crystals to altar tools—as well as a successful subscription-box series. Tamed Wild's popular blog, podcasts, readings, and retreats make it a leader in the earth-based magick marketplace. Shelby is a tarot reader, astrology lover, and past-life-regression practitioner. She lives in the Appalachian mountains with her husband, Jason, and is the mother of Chase and Saylor.

Kate Belew is a Brooklyn-based writer, poet, storyteller, and witch from Michigan. Her work spans genres and spaces: poetry, nonprofits, immersive theatre, health and wellness, herbalism, witchcraft, and the psychedelic. She cohosts *Magick & Alchemy*, a Tamed Wild podcast about mythology and witchcraft. Kate facilitates and teaches writing workshops and has an MFA in poetry from Sarah Lawrence College. Her writing can be found in a variety of publications, both digital and print.

Kate has studied herbalism with Chestnut School of Herbal Medicine online and Kathryn Solie's poisonous plants series, and through an apprenticeship with Green Witch Robin Rose Bennett—in addition to her life experience and self-study, in tandem with her love of books. Kate is a lifelong student of the plants, stars, and poetry.